The SAGES Manual
on the Fundamental Use
of Surgical Energy (FUSE)

D1561808

The SAGES Manual on the Fundamental Use of Surgical Energy (FUSE)

Liane S. Feldman, MD, FACS, FRCS(C)
McGill University Health Centre, Montreal, QC, Canada

Pascal R. Fuchshuber, MD, PhD, FACS
The Permanente Medical Group, Inc., Walnut Creek, CA, USA

Daniel B. Jones, MD, MS, FACS
Harvard Medical School, Beth Israel Deaconess Medical Center, Boston, MA, USA

Editors

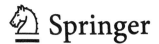 Springer

Editors
Liane S. Feldman, MD, FACS, FRCS(C)
McGill University Health Centre
Montreal, QC, Canada

Pascal R. Fuchshuber, MD, PhD, FACS
The Permanente Medical Group, Inc.
Walnut Creek, CA, USA

Daniel B. Jones, MD, MS, FACS
Harvard Medical School
Beth Israel Deaconess Medical Center
Boston, MA, USA

ISBN 978-1-4614-2073-6   e-ISBN 978-1-4614-2074-3
DOI 10.1007/978-1-4614-2074-3
Springer New York Dordrecht Heidelberg London

Library of Congress Control Number: 2011944511

Springer is part of Springer Science+Business Media (www.springer.com)

Foreword

Some things are not spoken about much in part because we would like to think they are rare events or we really, truly believe, "it could never happen to me." Yet, device misfires, accidental burns, and operating rooms fires do occur—more often than you'd think. And many times these adverse events are totally preventable.

The vast majority of surgical procedures in every specialty performed throughout the world involve the use of some device that applies energy to tissue. As such, there must be a standardized curriculum for surgeons (and perhaps allied health personnel) that addresses the physics, safe use, and complications associated with these devices that promotes the best outcomes for patients.

The SAGES Manual on the Fundamental Use of Surgical Energy is intended to serve as an easy to read companion to the FUSE online educational program/curriculum developed by the Society of American Gastrointestinal and Endoscopic Surgeons (SAGES). The chapters review the use of energy in the operating room and endoscopic procedure areas.

The general topics covered by the *The SAGES Manual on the Fundamental Use of Surgical Energy* include the physics of electrical energy applications, safe use of electrical, ultrasonic, and other forms of energy and electrical tools in the OR, recognition of faulty equipment and application of correct setting, and appropriate indications of energy tools and technology in the OR.

The SAGES Manual on the Fundamental Use of Surgical Energy is a comprehensive read of just about everything the practicing surgeon needs to know about surgical energy and devices. It should help prepare surgeons for the Self-Assessment Program for FUSE which leads to certification with a validated multiple choice test. The aim of the FUSE certificate will be to assure basic proficiency with basic didactic and specific tool based components.

Cambridge, MA, USA   *Steven D. Schwaitzberg, MD, FACS*
Boston, MA, USA   *Daniel B. Jones, MD, MS, FACS*

Introduction

How many different surgical energy devices are in your operating room today? Chances are you would have trouble coming up with a complete list. With increasing surgical specialization the number of energy devices has grown exponentially. Specifically designed devices exist for almost every surgical need using many different types of energy sources and designs. Often different devices compete for the same operative task. Many of today's surgical techniques and procedures owe their existence to these energy devices, and many of the future surgical innovations will depend on the development of new devices.

However, the introduction of new energy devices into surgical practice has occurred at a dizzying speed and essentially without any formal education about their safety and correct use. Surgeons who would firmly hold on to a specific type of suture material for their entire career can be seen readily switching to a new energy device with minimal or no instructions. Without the fundamental technical and safety knowledge about energy devices the surgeon puts himself at risk for injury to the patient and himself. There is a clear need for a curriculum on the safe and correct use of surgical energy devices.

This first edition of *The SAGES Manual on the Fundamental Use of Surgical Energy* tries to accomplish just that. It provides an educational tool for the practicing surgeon to acquire the necessary knowledge to use most currently available surgical energy devices. This Manual covers the fundamentals of electrical, ultrasonic, radiofrequency and microwave energy, their application in surgical devices and the appropriate use of these devices in adult and pediatric patients. It provides tips and guidance on how to manage the main safety issues related to energy devices in the OR such as fires, burn injuries, device failures, and interference with other medical devices.

The authors and editors have tried to avoid discussion of individual proprietary devices. As much as possible, we have tried to be generic and discuss fundamental principles. For figures and images, efforts were made to remove manufacturer's names and markings. When a specific device was included, attempts were made to include other devices of that type. Discussion of a device does not imply its endorsement by the authors, editors or SAGES.

The editors believe that *The SAGES Manual on the Fundamental Use of Surgical Energy* will become an indispensable tool for any surgeon or allied health professional wishing to enhance patient safety and efficiency in the use of surgical energy devices. The first 13 chapters of the manual provide fundamental knowledge to the safe use of these devices. The subsequent "enrichment" chapters allow the user to obtain a deeper understanding of the principles through hands-on simulations. Finally, a nomenclature for common terms related to electrosurgery and energy devices is included at the end. While readers may at first find it hard not to call for their "cautery", they will surely appreciate that the use of correct and consistent terminology is an important first step towards understanding the fundamental use of surgical energy. The FUSE manual is thus designed to be an integral part of the FUSE certification program developed by SAGES.

The editors would like to thank our expert faculty for their contributions, the outstanding SAGES staff (Jessica and Carla), and our supportive spouses (Hillel, Anne, and Stephanie).

Montreal, QC, Canada   *Liane S. Feldman, MD, FACS, FRCS(C)*
Walnut Creek, CA, USA   *Pascal R. Fuchshuber, MD, PhD, FACS*
Boston, MA, USA   *Daniel B. Jones, MD, MS, FACS*

Contents

Contributors

James G. Bittner IV, MD
Department of Surgery, Section of Minimally Invasive Surgery,
Washington University in St. Louis School of Medicine,
St. Louis, MO, USA

L. Michael Brunt, MD, FACS
Department of Surgery, Washington University School of Medicine,
St. Louis, MO, USA

James S. Choi, MD, FACS
Department of Surgery, The Permanente Medical Group, Inc.,
Walnut Creek, CA, USA

Brian J. Dunkin, MD, FACS
Weill Cornell Medical College, New York, NY, USA
The Methodist Hospital, The Methodist Institute for Technology,
Innovation, and Education (MITIE), Houston, TX, USA

Pascal R. Fuchshuber, MD, PhD, FACS
Hepatobiliary and Oncologic Surgery, The Permanente
Medical Group, Inc., Walnut Creek, CA, USA

Charlotte L. Guglielmi, MA, BSN, RN, CNOR
Beth Israel Deaconess Medical Center, Boston, MA, USA

Jeffrey W. Hazey, MD, FACS
Department of Surgery, The Ohio State University Medical Center,
Columbus, OH, USA

Daniel Herron, MD, FACS
Department of Surgery, The Mount Sinai Hospital,
New York, NY, USA

David A. Iannitti, MD, FACS
Department of Surgery, Carolinas Medical Center, Charlotte, NC, USA

Stephanie B. Jones, MD
Department of Anesthesia, Critical Care and Pain Medicine,
Beth Israel Deaconess Medical Center, Boston, MA, USA

Calvin D. Lyons, MD
The Methodist Hospital, The Methodist Institute for Technology,
Innovation, and Education (MITIE), Houston, TX, USA

Dean Mikami, MD, FACS
Department of Gastrointestinal Surgery, The Ohio State University
Medical Center, Columbus, OH, USA

Malcolm G. Munro, MD, FACOG, FRCS(c)
Department of Obstetrics and Gynecology, David Geffen School
of Medicine at UCLA, Los Angeles, CA, USA
Department of Obstetrics and Gynecology, Kaiser Permanente,
Los Angeles Medical Center, Los Angeles, CA, USA

Chan W. Park, MD
Department of Surgery, Duke University Medical Center,
Durham, NC, USA

Dana D. Portenier, MD, FACS
Department of Surgery, Duke University Medical Center,
Durham, NC, USA

Gretchen Purcell Jackson, MD, PhD, FACS
Department of Pediatric Surgery, Monroe Carell Jr. Children's
Hospital at Vanderbilt, Nashville, TN, USA

Marc A. Rozner, MD, PhD
Department of Anesthesiology and Perioperative Medicine, Department
of Cardiology, The University of Texas MD Anderson Cancer Center,
Houston, TX, USA

Steven D. Schwaitzberg, MD, FACS
Department of Surgery, Cambridge Health Alliance,
Harvard Medical School, Cambridge, MA, USA

Ryan Z. Swan, MD
Department of Surgery, Carolinas Medical Center,
Charlotte, NC, USA

J. Esteban Varela, MD, MPH, FACS
Department of Surgery, Section of Minimally Invasive
and Bariatric Surgery, Washington University School of Medicine,
St. Louis, MO, USA

C. Randle Voyles, MD, MS, FACS
University of Mississippi Medical Center, Jackson, MS, USA

Part I
Fundamentals of Surgical Energy

1. Evolutions and Revolutions in Surgical Energy

Steven D. Schwaitzberg

There is an unquestionable need for an organized surgical curriculum concerned with the application of energy in the surgical or endoscopic field. This is driven by a number of factors that are evolving rapidly, not the least of which are the technological choices themselves which are addressed in detail throughout this manual. The Fundamental Use of Surgical Energy (FUSE) represents an opportunity to address the changes brought about by the interactions of the *evolutions and revolutions* in technology, patient safety, surgical training, credentialing, and societal expectations.

Technology Evolutions/Revolutions

Energy has been applied in some form to tissue since the beginning of recorded history. Thermal cautery, the original application of surgical energy, was used for thousands of years essentially unchanged as the sole energy tool available to the early surgeons. Cautery is the application of energy as heat to tissues. This leads to tissue destruction and was invaluable as a method of controlling hemorrhage. The energy was transferred from fire to cauters (Fig. 1.1), which were fashioned in variety of shapes and sizes for application. The temperature of the cauters could range from 400°C visible as red heat in the dark to 1,000°C seen as bright cherry red. Clearly, a certain amount of expertise (training?) must have been needed to master the very heating of the cauter to achieve no more than a dull red glow in order to avoid unnecessary tissue damage. The uses of cautery can be traced as early as the Neolithic period where recovered skulls show evidences of cauterization. Indian writings from 2000 BC suggest cautery was used to destroy breast lesions.

L.S. Feldman et al. (eds.), *The SAGES Manual on the Fundamental Use of Surgical Energy (FUSE)*, DOI 10.1007/978-1-4614-2074-3_1, © Springer Science+Business Media, LLC 2012

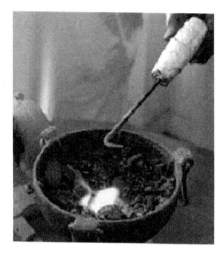

Fig. 1.1. Cauter being heated in open fire.

Hippocrates approximately 500 BC is said to have favored cautery as a treatment to destroy lesions when other methods failed. Uses have been varied through the ages including hemostasis, tumor destruction, branding, and it was even used to open short segment imperforate anus. Ancient Chinese used a form of cautery known as moxabustion where the moxa herb is burned, on or near the skin at a location determined by the condition that was intended to be treated. The application of cautery as the primary modality to treat traumatic vessel hemorrhage was finally challenged by the work of Ambrose Pare who demonstrated the superiority of the simple ligature in the 1550s. The application of cautery has not been abandoned in modern medicine. The fire heated cauter has evolved into a variety of instruments such as small battery powered cautery instruments used in many emergency departments to drain subungual hematomas (Fig. 1.2) or augment minor surgery.

The electrical revolution in surgery had its roots with early work in the late 1800s and early 1900s by Morton, d'Arsonval, Nagelschmidt, Pozzi, Rivere, Doyen, and Clark and has proceeded with an accelerating pace over the last 100 years. This initial work was primarily centered on fulguration of tumors. The first volley of the modern era was fired by William Bovie and Harvey Cushing. William T. Bovie (1882–1958) (Fig. 1.3) began his academic career as a botanist and did his graduate work in plant physiology at Harvard. He then remained at Harvard to work for the Cancer Commission where he developed interest in

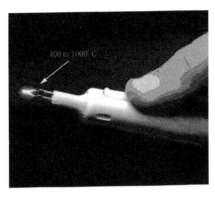

Fig. 1.2. Battery powered ophthalmologic eye cautery. Local tip temperatures can exceed 1,000°C.

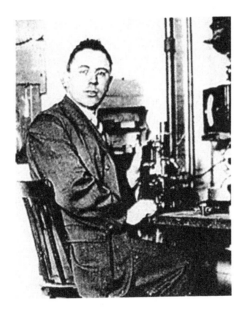

Fig. 1.3. Willim T. Bovie, PhD.

electrosurgery. While others had already developed the concepts of spark gap generators for fulguration and low voltage waveform generators for cutting, Dr Bovie was the first to develop an electrosurgical unit that provided both cutting and coagulation settings and added an instrument

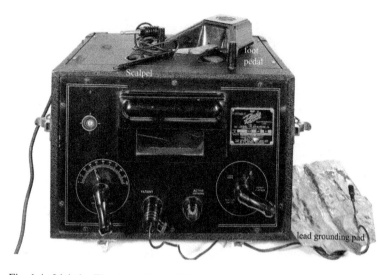

Fig. 1.4. Liebel—Flarsheim "Bovie." The unit was used in the mid 1930s. Note the lead grounding pad and reusable handpiece. (From the collection of John Abele, with permission).

that was hand-held via a pistol grip, allowing for hand activation and interchangeable electrodes. Harvey Cushing, the father of modern neurosurgery, contemplated operative uses of electrosurgery as early as 1925. However, it was in 1926, when the removal of a brain tumor had to be abandoned due to excessive vascularity that one of his residents suggested he reattempt excision using the electrosurgical loop cutting tool developed by Dr Bovie. On October 1, 1926 Dr Cushing successfully removed the remainder of the tumor. Clinical electrosurgery was born. Electrosurgical units are still commonly referred to as "the Bovie" by most surgeons today. Today's entrepreneurs would be disappointed to learn that Dr Bovie never financially profited from his invention having reportedly sold his patent to the Liebel-Flarsheim Co, for the princely sum of $1.00.in the 1920s. They produced "Bovie" electrosurgical units (Fig. 1.4) as well as other devices such as short wave diathermy units (Fig. 1.5). Other early devices utilized Tesla coils with exposed spark gap generators (imagine the fire risk) (Fig. 1.6). The Birtcher Crusader introduced in the late 1930s was the forerunner to the "hyfrecator" (hyfrequency eradicator) which was commonly used in awake patients in office settings (Fig. 1.7). They utilized low power, allowing the patient to become the capacitor and current sink without the need for a grounding pad. The devices worked through *dessication*—tissues destruction from

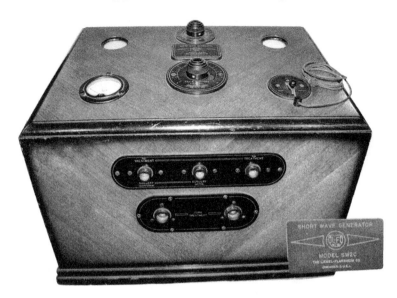

Fig. 1.5. Liebel Flarsheim short wave radiofrequency generators used in the 1930s. (From the collection of John Abele, with permission).

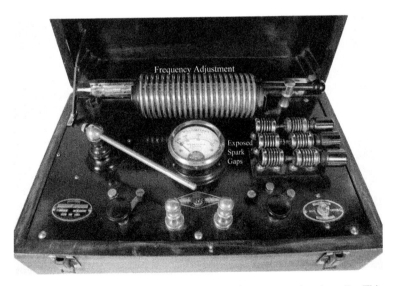

Fig. 1.6. McIntosh diathermy with adjustable frequency and tesla coils. This unit was produced in the late 1920s. This featured exposed spark gaps generators (Tesla coil) and adjustable frequency generation. (From the collection of John Abele, with permission).

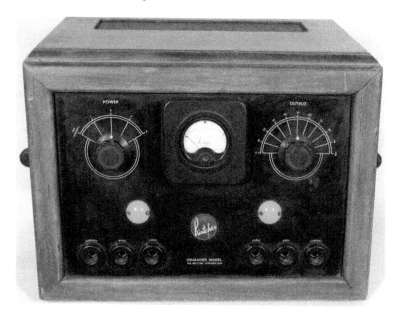

Fig. 1.7. Birtcher Crusader developed in the 1930s. (From the collection of John Abele, with permission).

the heat generated at the tip of the handpiece or *fulgaration* by intentionally sparking the tissue thus generating extremely high tissue temperature at the point of entry leading to tissue *carbonization*.

Following his early work with two point coagulation electrosurgery. Electrosurgery with bipolar instruments was introduced in neurosurgery during the 1940s by James Greenwood at Methodist Hospital in Houston, Texas. This device still required a grounding pad. This concept was subsequently modified by Leonard Malis (Fig. 1.8), a neurosurgeon at Mount Sinai in New York, into the bipolar device as we know it today with current flowing between the two electrodes of the bipolar instrument. This was developed into a commercially available device in 1955. Bipolar electrosurgical instrumentation for gynecology was developed in 1973 by the Canadian gynecologist and noted laparoscopist Jacques Emile-Rioux (Fig. 1.9). His ingenuity arose out of frustration associated with intestinal injury caused by monopolar instrumentation used for electrosurgery during tubal sterilization. He envisioned placing the second return electrode within the instrument itself rather than placed remotely as a dispersive electrode. He built an alpha prototype at home from coat hangers and a broom handle. The university electrical

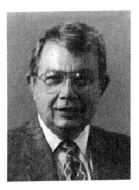

Fig. 1.8. Leonard Malis, MD.

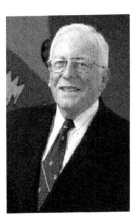

Fig. 1.9. Jacques Emile-Rioux.

engineering department built a beta prototype a week later. Almost impossible to do today, he then took this homemade device into the operating room where he used a monopolar instrument on one tube and the prototypical bipolar device on the other during a hysterectomy. Histological examination revealed sufficient tubal destruction by the bipolar device without the significant lateral spread seen in the tube coagulated with the monopolar instrument. Despite the fact that coagulation with a bipolar instrument is slower compared to that of a monopolar device, bipolar instruments quickly became a common modality in gynecologic surgery, neurosurgery, and microsurgery. Development of bipolar instrumentation has continued to this day with newer devices used by a variety of specialties especially in the arena of minimally invasive surgery where cutting blades have been incorporated into the device. In addition, newer devices incorporate real time measurement of tissue impedance that allows the system to alert the surgeon when the tissue between the jaws of the device is no longer conductive because it has been completely coagulated.

In 1994, Joseph Amaral reported the results of experimental studies using ultrasonically generated vibration as a source of mechanical energy to heat, seal, and divide tissue. A transducer in the handpiece vibrates at very high frequencies (around 23,000 to 55,000 times per second) which is translated through the shaft of the device to the contiguous blade or jaw grasping the tissue where the protein is heated to 60°C and denatured. If a grasping type design is used to compress a vessel, the resulting coagulum effectuates a secure vessel seal. The ultrasonic coagulator became a key enabling and revolutionary technology in the early days of advanced minimally invasive surgery pushing forward the development of procedures like laparoscopic Nissen fundoplication, adrenalectomy, and splenectomy. Today, this has evolved into a variety of open and laparoscopic ultrasonic coagulation devices.

Evolutions and Revolutions in Credentialing

For at least the last 3 decades, freshly minted graduate surgeons who came to hospitals to practice filled out a list of procedures according to self-assessed competency. It was generally expected that the Chief of Surgery would sign off on just about whatever was checked off. Today, considering most surgical disciplines, specialization has increasingly become the rule, especially in the urban setting.

The nature of referral patterns, fellowships, and competitive opportunities has become the driver of the types of operations the surgeon performs. Certainly, there is a body of literature that supports some (perhaps imperfect) relationship between case volume and clinical outcome. The net result is that service chiefs are subjecting surgical privilege requests to increasing scrutiny, fearful that allowing a surgeon to perform case types on an infrequent basis may cause patient harm and perhaps even derivative liability to the chief/hospital. The Joint Commission revolutionized this process when, beginning on January 1, 2010, competency assessment was required upon arrival to the medical staff (focused professional practice evaluation—FPPE) and on an ongoing basis (ongoing professional practice evaluation—OPPE).

It is safe to say that determining procedural competency is challenging. Objective measures are difficult to develop beyond hemorrhage, infection, ICU admission, and return to the operating room, all of which are adverse outcomes. Evidence of training and ongoing continuing medical education that is relevant to practice have become constructive elements of competency assessment. For example, the movement to reduce central line infection has demonstrated astounding success through team training, part of which is mandatory operator education on the prevention of infection and line insertion techniques. In many hospitals, the privilege of central line insertion is not granted unless this education is completed successfully.

Should this mandatory educational process be applied to surgical energy devices? It is becoming clear that residency training alone will be insufficient to prepare a surgeon for practice and that surgeons will have to provide evidence of the completion of specific curricula before being allowed to perform a variety of procedures. Up until now, there has been no established training curriculum in surgical energy consistently applied across surgical training programs. Is one needed? The counter argument to yet another required course of education is that surgeons become expert because some form of energy is used on nearly every case, which is often offered as a "competency-by-osmosis" approach to education. If this were truly effective, then the devastating injuries from OR fires, thermal burns, and visceral perforations would not occur. Furthermore, there is no guarantee that the same devices used in training will be available in the hospital where one establishes one's practice.

Where does this leave the plethora of energy devices available to the surgeon? Most hospitals require a specific training program for laser use but not for radiofrequency, ultrasonic, hyperthermal, microwave, or cryotherapeutic instrumentation. Even if required who would/should provide or pay for this education- the surgeon who uses the device, the hospital that bought the device, or the company that sold the device? Continuous declines in provider reimbursement will challenge the creation and funding of this education. At the same time, the current trends in many states and institutions to severely limit industry–physician contact will significantly hamper some of the more positive aspects of these interactions in terms of device education and training.

The FUSE program was created to fill the gaps created by these multiple simultaneously moving forces. There is a clear mandate for independent production of educational materials, but in the case of energy device education and training this must be developed in a transparent partnership with the device industry in order to create a scientifically accurate and clinically relevant program in energy and energy device education for surgical teams across a wide spectrum of specialties. Certainly, the surgeon in any specialty who can present credentials of successful training and assessment for specific energy devices, even from residency, simplifies the issue of privileges for service chiefs and OR managers.

There are plenty of parallels in other industries. The multidisciplinary approach to FUSE recognizes that safe surgical energy application requires a team approach to achieve optimal performance. Each member of the surgical team needs to be aware of all of the pitfalls that may result in suboptimal performance or a complication. As a result well-executed procedures are team successes, but the whole team must also own the failures or poor results. The surgeon must become the master of his/her tools from setup through the procedure all the way to device breakdown. Conversely, the operating room nurse must be able to recognize potentially unsafe situations of energy application during the operative aspects of the procedure. The FUSE program will allow surgical teams to achieve a higher level of common understanding regarding surgical energy by establishing a defined knowledge base and a set of assessment tools.

Evolution and Revolutions in Societal Expectations

It was not that long ago that patients were simply referred to a surgeon by their doctors and it was taken on faith that the referral was a good one. The revolution that has marked the Internet age has placed more information (both accurate and inaccurate) in the hands of patients. Similarly, the mandatory public reporting of outcomes for a wide variety of measures has impacted the referral process significantly. Patients are now looking for information that their surgeon is associated with good outcomes.

Does this bar define competency or something higher? Today's patients are searching for expertise whenever they can. Consider the airline industry. Passengers get onboard the aircraft and entrust their lives to the skill of the pilot. What are the assumptions? They expect the copilot to be competent, however society demands that the captain is a truly skilled individual who can handle a wide variety of situations and operate all aspects of the aircraft necessary to bring the plane safely to the ground. When an aircraft is upgraded with a new piece of technology, the flight crew is trained in its use. If it is fundamentally different, such as when GPS (global positioning system) navigation technology was introduced to replace the older VOR (variable frequency omnidirectional-radiorange) systems, the theory and physics of operation are included in the education plan. Simulation is often used to verify competency prior to using it in flight. Simulation also allows the pilot to be exposed to uncommon scenarios that would take a long time to accumulate. A passenger never walks onto the plane wondering if the pilot knows how to work all of the instruments new and old—it is simply expected.

The patient who undergoes a surgical procedure gives up a certain amount of autonomy especially when procedures are performed under general anesthesia. He/she expects us to safely operate the devices used inside their body. What does this mean? Are we supposed to be able to personally build or repair these devices? Neither a bus driver nor a pilot can repair the engine of their vehicle, yet both are expected to recognize situations when proceeding with travel might be dangerous or deal with unusual situations. It is reasonable to expect that every member of the surgical team should be able to set up the energy devices to be used in a procedure, recognize when the device is not working properly, troubleshoot the user-controllable aspects of the device and operate them safely within the body. Such a skill set requires training by all members of the surgical team. It is unlikely that a truly well-informed patient would let a surgeon use a surgical energy device on them if the competency if not the expertise using that tool could not be established. How would a patient feel if the nurse had never set it up before? Think about it the next time you need a procedure. Should we expect less from our patients?

Summary

While revolutionary in concept, the FUSE program itself will grow to accommodate more devices and more technologies over time. By building a scalable framework, our understanding, competency, and expertise in the use of surgical energy will evolve in a synchronous fashion with the technology.

2. Fundamentals of Electrosurgery Part I: Principles of Radiofrequency Energy for Surgery

Malcolm G. Munro

Electrosurgery is the use of radiofrequency (RF) alternating current (AC) to raise intracellular temperature in order to achieve vaporization or the combination of desiccation and protein coagulation. These effects can be translated into cutting or coagulation of tissue, the latter usually to attain hemostasis, but also to occlude lumen-containing structures, or to destroy large volumes of tissue such as soft tissue neoplasms. The concept of RF electrosurgery must be distinguished clearly from the process of cautery, derived from the Greek *kauterion* (hot iron), in which the destruction or denaturation of tissue is by the passive transfer of heat from a heated instrument. In short, RF electrosurgery is *not* cautery.

Electrical energy has been used in the performance of surgical procedures since the late nineteenth century. However, it wasn't until the introduction of the first electrosurgical generator (or electrosurgical unit) (ESU) by Bovie as reported in 1928 that the potential of RF electrosurgery was popularized [1]. Similar to any surgical procedure or instrument, RF electricity was found to have its own unique issues that resulted in unanticipated complications. Since that time, much has been learned about the biophysics involved in the use of RF electricity, and both devices and techniques have evolved to the point where the energy can be applied safely and effectively. However, to do so, it is necessary for the surgeon to possess an understanding of the fundamentals of RF alternating current, and the impacts of RF electricity on tissue, and the mechanisms whereby adverse outcomes can occur.

L.S. Feldman et al. (eds.), *The SAGES Manual on the Fundamental Use of Surgical Energy (FUSE)*, DOI 10.1007/978-1-4614-2074-3_2, © Springer Science+Business Media, LLC 2012

History of Electrosurgery

The use of heat for the treatment of wounds can be traced to Neolithic times [2]. Ancient Egyptians (*c.* 3000 BC) have described the use of thermal cautery to treat ulcers and tumors of the breast, Hippocrates (469–370 BC) employed heat to destroy a neck tumor, and Albucasis (*c.* 980) was reported to have used a hot iron to control bleeding [3, 4]. Direct current (DC) was the first electrical energy used for medical therapeutics, first described in the mid-eighteenth century by contemporary scientists such as Benjamin Franklin and John Wesley. Indeed the techniques used relied on the use of DC to heat an instrument that was then applied to tissue causing a tissue effect secondary to *passive* heat transfer. The resulting coagulation and desiccation of the tissue was, and is, a form of cautery [5].

In the latter part of the nineteenth century, investigators in Europe and the United States began experimenting with the biological effects of *AC* on tissue. One of the pioneers was Arsené D'Arsonval, a French inventor and physiologist, who, in 1893, was the first to report these effects used in a clinical context [6]. He designed capacitors, later modified by Oudlin, which developed a high-voltage discharge in the form of sparks that could arc to, and superficially destroy nearby tissue, a process termed *fulguration* (from the Latin noun *fulgur* for lightening, and the verb *fulgurare*, to flash).

In 1907, Rivère, a student of D'Arsonval, demonstrated that if high-frequency AC was applied directly to tissue, without sparking, another electrosurgical process called "white coagulation" occurred [7]. Shortly thereafter, in 1909, Doyen described the use of bipolar RF instruments for the coagulation of tissue [8]. In the next 10–20 years, more powerful generators allowed these techniques to be employed in humans to treat nevi, granulation tissue, and bladder tumors.

An important step in the development of electrosurgery was de Forest's invention, in 1907, of the "Audion" (US Patent 879,532) a triode-containing vacuum tube that amplified electrical signals and served as the lynchpin for radio broadcasting. Coincidentally, of course, the invention also facilitated production of the types of high-frequency continuous AC necessary to evenly coagulate, or, if properly focused, to vaporize tissue. Linear propagation of vaporization would result in tissue transection or cutting. In 1924 Wyeth became the first to report use of a vacuum tube-generated, continuous alternating RF current to cut tissue in humans [9].

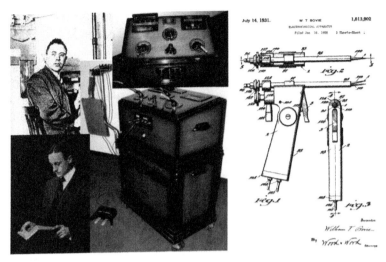

Fig. 2.1. Historical collage. William T. Bovie (*upper left*) was the inventor of the electrosurgical generator. The machine coupled a spark gap generator (for high-voltage modulated outputs) and a generator producing a continuous low-voltage waveform (*upper and lower middle panels*). The patent and a diagram of the pistol gripped monopolar instrument are shown on the *right*. It allowed for rapid changing of the electrodes. The famed neurosurgeon Harvey W. Cushing (*lower left*) was the first to use the instrument in 1926 demonstrating the remarkable ability to reduce intraoperative hemorrhage. From that point on the perioperative morbidity and mortality associated with intracranial surgery dramatically decreased.

While Bovie, a physicist, and Cushing, a neurosurgeon, are often given credit for the invention of electrosurgery, they were actually only its most effective early promoters (Fig. 2.1). In 1926, Cushing used Bovie's side-by-side ESUs—one, a vacuum tube-based design for cutting, the other, a spark gap version for coagulation—to perform neurosurgery on a patient with an otherwise inoperable vascular myeloma. The results of this and other procedures were published in 1928 [1]. While there are important differences, the original "Bovie" machine served as the model for virtually all subsequently produced electrosurgical units (ESUs) until the invention of solid-state generators and isolated circuits in the 1970s. The principal advantage of such generators is that they can produce lower voltage, and more consistent waveforms while their isolated circuitry allows for the creation and use of systems designed to improve safety, such as impedance monitoring.

It may be a surprise to some that endoscopically directed electro-surgery was first performed as early as 1910. Kelly describes Beer's use of a monopolar instrument to fulgurate bladder tumors under cystoscopic guidance [7]. One of the first attempts at using laparoscopically directed electrosurgery was reported by Fervers, a general surgeon, who in 1933 described electrosurgical adhesiolysis [10]. Several years later, in 1941, Power and Barnes reported the first reported human performance of laparoscopic electrosurgical female sterilization using a monopolar instrument [11].

In the 1970s and early 1980s, there was widespread belief that activated unipolar laparoscopic instruments could arc long and variable distances to adjacent viscera causing significant thermal injury. However, in 1985, Levy and Soderstrom demonstrated that under reasonable conditions, such injuries were infrequent, and that almost all the purported bowel injuries were indeed secondary to physical, not electrical trauma. (It is likely that most or all of these injuries were caused by insertion of trocar cannula systems [12]). In addition, there developed a better understanding of the risks presented by the use of high power outputs (up to 600 W) and the factors, such as "capacitive coupling," that contribute to electrosurgical complications. Since that time, safety has been further enhanced by newer generators with isolated circuits and monitoring systems for the early detection of separation of the dispersive or electrode from the patient.

The concerns around unipolar instrumentation contributed to the further development and popularization of laparoscopic bipolar instruments in the early 1970s by Frangenheim and Rioux [13, 14]. These designs were used essentially unchanged until the early twenty-first century, when a number of proprietary bipolar systems emerged based on the recognition that RF-electrosurgical coagulation and desiccation could be used to predictably seal vessels of substantial size, and with much reduced lateral thermal injury.

RF electrosurgery has now become widely accepted as a highly effective method of cutting and obtaining hemostasis. Bipolar instruments offer some safety advantages when used for the processes of coagulation and desiccation but are in general not useful for cutting or vaporization. Safe and effective application of either requires the use of well-designed equipment and a sound understanding of electrosurgical principles.

Principles of Electrosurgery

With the advent of surgical lasers, institutional credentialing committees ensured that surgeons clearly demonstrated knowledge of laser physics prior to allowing them to use the equipment in their facilities. Unfortunately, such rigorous requirements have not, to date, been applied to electrosurgery. Consequently, generations of physicians have had extensive experience with an instrument that most do not understand, a factor that likely contributed significantly to the incidence of RF electricity-related surgical complications. Like all energy sources, RF electricity should be respected, not feared. However, for safe and effective use, it is mandatory that the surgeon possess a clear understanding of the principles of electrosurgery.

During RF electrosurgery, the electromagnetic energy is converted in the cells first to kinetic energy then to thermal energy. The desired effect in the tissue is determined by a number of electrical properties as well as factors such as tissue exposure time and the size and shape of the surface of the electrode near to or in contact with the target tissue.

So what is "alternating current?" The answer starts with a description of the requirements for an electrical circuit. For any electrical circuit to exist, there must be a positive and negative pole to create the conditions for movement of ions and/or electrons. In a *DC*, the polarity in the circuit remains constant, as does the flow of the electrons (Fig. 2.2a). Common everyday examples of DC circuits are found wherever the power source is a battery, like a flashlight. When the polarity switches back and forth, which is the case for standard "wall outlet" sources, the term *AC* is used, a circumstance that reflects the alternating polarity of the circuit (Fig. 2.2b).

In North American outlets, the polarity of the output changes 60 times per second, or 60 Hz. This frequency allows us to power our homes and appliances, but also has the ability to depolarize muscle and neural cells as will be discussed later in this chapter. However, if the frequency of the polar change is increased dramatically, in excess of 100,000 Hz, or 100 kHz, the muscles and nerves cannot respond and, in essence, function normally. Furthermore, such frequencies can be used surgically to impact the cells and tissue in a dramatically effective fashion. Because the frequencies typically used for surgery are around 500 KHz, the frequency of amplitude modification (AM) radio broadcasts, the term RF electrosurgery is used (Fig. 2.3).

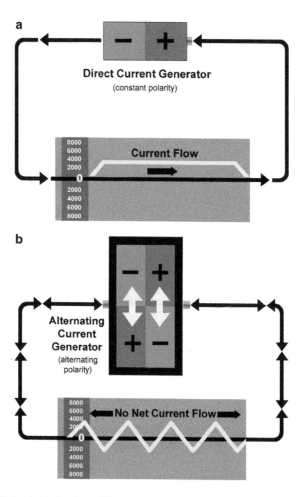

Fig. 2.2. (**a**, **b**) Direct vs. Alternating current. The *upper panel* depicts an electrical circuit created by an energy source with constant polarity, a battery, with the resultant unidirectional flow of electrons. The oscilloscope reflects the output with a constant deflection on one side of the "0" line. In the *bottom panel*, the energy source is an alternating current with each pole constantly switching from negative to positive, and a waveform that spends equal amounts of time above and below "0." As a result, there is no directional flow—the electrons can be perceived to be oscillating, not flowing. This should explain why the term "return" does not apply to alternating current circuits.

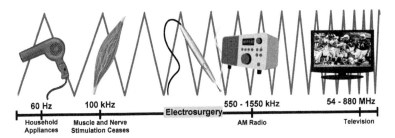

60 Hz	100 kHz		550 - 1550 kHz	54 - 880 MHz
		Electrosurgery		
Household Appliances	Muscle and Nerve Stimulation Ceases		AM Radio	Television

Fig. 2.3. Electromagnetic spectrum. Wavelength shortens as frequency increases. Wall outlets provide a waveform with a frequency of 50–60 Hz (cycles per second). Radiofrequency starts at about 300,000 Hz or 300 KHz and extends through about 3 MHz (3×10^6 Hz). In this frequency neither muscular nor neural cells depolarize.

As with any electrical process, RF electrosurgery requires the creation of an electrical circuit that includes the two electrodes, the patient, the ESU, and the connecting wires (Fig. 2.4). All contemporary RF electrosurgery is "bipolar" for it is necessary to have two electrodes; what differs is the location and purpose of the second electrode (Fig. 2.4). Bipolar *instruments* have both electrodes mounted on the device, usually located on or near to the distal end so that only the tissue located between the two electrodes is included in the circuit. However, with *unipolar instruments* only one electrode is mounted on the device and the entire patient is interposed between this "active electrode" and the large dispersive electrode that is also attached to the ESU, but located relatively distant from the target tissue, typically on the thigh or back. The narrow active electrode concentrates the current (and therefore the power), at the designated site, elevating the intracellular temperature, while the dispersive electrode acts as the other pole, "processing" the same amount of current (and power), but dispersing it over the entirety of the large surface area, so much so that the temperature in the underlying skin does not rise, thereby preventing tissue injury.

The three interacting properties of electricity that affect the temperature rise in tissue are current (I), voltage (V), and impedance or resistance (R) (Table 2.1). (The rational for use of the letter "I" for current likely relates to the French inventor-scientist Ampere who used the term *intensité* to describe the intensity of flow when describing what we now know as an electrical current. Consequently, the letter "I" was adopted by Ohm and others when describing current.) Current is a measure of the electron movement across or past a point in the circuit in a given period

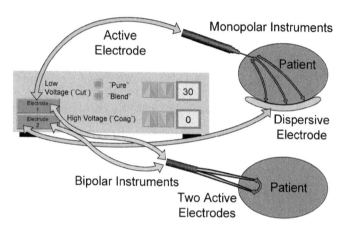

All RF Electrosurgery is "Bipolar"
Monopolar vs Bipolar Instrumentation

Fig. 2.4. All radiofrequency electrosurgery is "bipolar," it is the location and purpose of the second electrode that varies. Monopolar instruments are used in monopolar systems (*top*). One of the two electrodes in such systems is designed to concentrate the current/power to achieve a surgical effect ("active" electrode), while the second electrode is placed remotely on the patient to disperse the current ("dispersive" electrode) thereby preventing the elevation of tissue temperature. Monopolar systems include the entire patient in the circuit, a circumstance that offers the opportunity for current diversion. Bipolar systems include both electrodes in the hand instrument (*bottom*). In most (but not all) instances, both electrodes are of small enough surface area to act as "active" electrodes thereby creating a surgical effect. In some instances, the electrode on the instrument serves as a dispersive electrode (see Figs. 2.2–2.13). The only part of the patient involved in the circuit is that adjacent to the electrodes, a circumstance that makes current diversion a virtual impossibility. Note that the same generator can usually support both systems (see also Fig. 2.7).

of time. It is measured in *amperes*. Voltage describes the electrical differential created between two points in a circuit that determines with what pressure the electrons are "pushed" within the circuit, including the parts of the circuit that comprise tissue. It is measured in *volts*. Resistance is measured in *ohms*, and is a reflection of the difficulty a given substance (e.g., tissue or the composition of the electrical wires) presents to the passage of electrons. The term resistance is generally reserved for DC while for AC, the term *impedance* is generally used. In a given circuit,

Table 2.1. Definitions of variables commonly used in the description of RF electrosurgery that can impact effect on cells and tissue.

Variable	Definition	Units
Current (I)	Flow of electrons past a point in the circuit/unit time	Amperes (coulombs/second)
Voltage (V)	Difference in electrical potential between two points in the circuit; force required to push a charge along the circuit	Volts (joules/coulomb)
Impedance (resistance) (R)	Degree to which the circuit or a portion of the circuit impedes the flow of electrons	Ohms
Power (P)	Work; amount of energy per unit time. Product of V and I	Watts (joules/second)
Energy	Capacity of a force to do work; cannot be created or destroyed	Joules (watts/second)

Table 2.2. Equations useful for the understanding of RF electrosurgical principles and calculation of impact on tissue.

Variable	Equation	Units
Ohm's law	Current $I = V/R$	Amperes (coulombs/second)[a]
	Voltage $V = I/R$	Volts (joules/coulomb)
	Impedance $R = V/I$	Ohms
Power (P)	$P = V \times I$	Watts (joules/second)
	$P = V \times V/R = V^2/R$	Watts (joules/second)
	$P = I \times I/R = I^2/R$	Watts (joules/second)
Energy (Q)	$Q = P \times t$ (second)	Joules (watts/second)

[a] A coulomb is the charge transferred by a current of 1 A for 1 s

these properties are related by *Ohm's law*—$I = V/R$ first described by Georg Ohm in 1827 [15] (Table 2.2).

An effective hydraulic analogy explaining Ohm's law has been designed by Roger Odell. The height of the water tower above the ground creates a pressure differential that can then be exerted upon the water in the outflow pipe (Fig. 2.5). This pressure differential can be analogized to voltage—the higher the tower, and that on the ground the greater the pressure differential between that on the water in the tower. When the spigot is opened, the water is allowed to flow, a process that is analogous to activating an electrical circuit (turning it on). (For DC this analogy is sound, but for AC, the flow actually oscillates back and forth with the

24   M.G. Munro

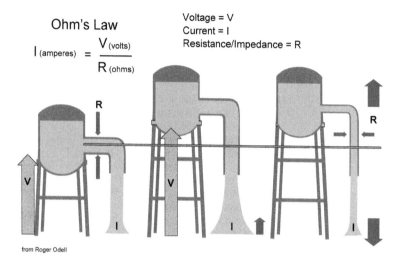

from Roger Odell

Fig. 2.5. Hydraulic analogy to explain Ohm's law. The height of the water tower serves as a surrogate for voltage (*V*)—a pressure differential between two points in a circuit. The amount of water that flows through the spigot per unit time represents current (*I*). The resistance or impedance to the flow of water is represented by the diameter of the spigot (*R*). If the voltage is increased (increasing the height of the water tower) and the impedance is held constant, current will increase proportionately (*middle*). If the voltage is held constant, and impedance increased, current will decrease. This is the reason for standard ESUs to lose efficiency when they encounter highly impedant tissue. Newer generators sense the increased impedance and increase the voltage thereby keeping power constant. To apply this concept to a RF output, imagine that it depicts what is happening during the course of about 1/500,000th of a second.

changing polarity of the generator, a fact that has to be considered when understanding this analogous situation.) The width of the spigot or pipe has a direct effect on the amount of water that can flow and, consequently, is analogous to the terms "resistance" and "impedance." If widened (reducing impedance), flow would be increased because there is reduced resistance to the flow of water. Electrosurgical resistance or impedance is impacted by a number of factors throughout the circuit, but, most importantly, by tissue characteristics. Hydrated tissue that contains ions has the lowest impedance, while dehydrated (desiccated) tissue or any tissue with lower ionic content (such as scarred tissue or fat) will have higher impedance and provide increased resistance to the flow of the current just as the narrow pipe in our water tower analogy reduces the rate of flow of the water from the tower.

Another important equation to the understanding RF electrosurgery is that which defines the relationship between voltage (V), current, (I), and power (W). Power in effect is a measure of work per unit time $(W = V \times I)$. If Ohm's Law is used to substitute for current (I), then power in watts can be expressed in another way: $[W = V(V/R)]$ or $(W = V^2/R)$. This demonstrates that power rises exponentially with increases in voltage and decreases inversely with increases in resistance or impedance.

These relationships are helpful in explaining a number of features of RF electrosurgery. For example, the ratio of voltage to current is largely responsible for the differing effects on tissue, given similar electrode size and shape as well as tissue exposure time. In general, the "pressure" of increased voltage enhances the ability of the current to arc from the electrode to tissue when there is a gap between them. When there is contact between the electrode and tissue, increased voltage forces more energy into the tissue, a circumstance that generally fosters a deeper or larger amount of thermal injury. The second equation shows how, at a given ESU output in watts, the voltage in the circuit will diminish if the tissue resistance increases, a feature that also decreases the power output from the ESU. This helps to explain how the cutting or coagulating characteristics of an electrode may change as tissues with different resistance are encountered. Newer ESUs can measure the impedance in tissue, and, as it rises or falls, can vary the voltage to maintain the output to be consistent with the desired power setting.

Perhaps the most important concept for the surgeon is that of power or current density, for control of this variable is what governs the impact of RF energy on tissue. It can be analogized the use of a magnifying glass to focus the power from a defined area of sunlight to one point, a process used by children for centuries to thermally carve one's initials into a piece of wood, or by campers to start a fire (Fig. 2.6). Simply put, current density is the amount of current per unit area; power density is simply proportional to the square of current density. Very high current density concentrated at the tip of an electrode can be used to heat and vaporize cells, slightly lower current density may desiccate and coagulate, while the same current spread over a large area may have no impact on the cells, the circumstance created by the design of a dispersive electrode.

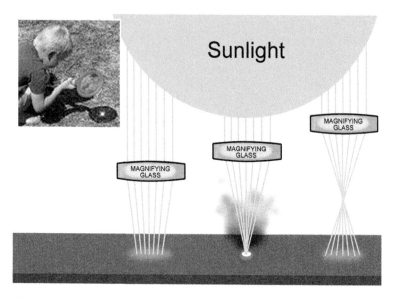

Fig. 2.6. Current/power density. RF electrosurgery is basically the control of power density, or current density and the sites of interface between the electrodes and the tissue. It can be analogized to the use of a magnifying glass, sunlight, and a wooden surface. If the light is kept relatively defocused (*right* and *left*) temperature in the wood does not increase, but if the light, and therefore the electromagnetic energy, is focused adequately (*middle*) the temperature of the wood increases to the point that it can burn.

Electrosurgical Generators

The ESU converts the low-frequency AC from a wall outlet (60 Hz in North America) into higher-voltage RF output, typically from 300 to 500 kHz (Fig. 2.7). Such ESUs are also capable of producing a number of different waveforms that allow the surgeon to change the impact of the energy on the targeted tissue. Features of the ESU output can be displayed on an oscilloscope (Fig. 2.8). The wave is generally symmetrical above and below "0" volts reflecting the continuously alternating polarity inherent to an AC. While the peak voltage generated is calculated by measuring the distance from the baseline to the apex of the wave, outputs are typically reported as the voltage differential between a peak and a trough or the "peak-to-peak" voltage. This image of the oscillating wave, below and above 0 V, should help the reader

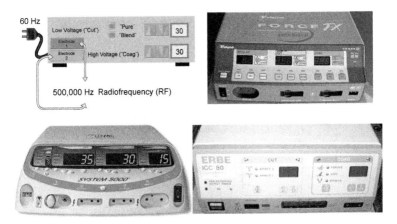

Fig. 2.7. A stylized electrosurgical unit (ESU) is depicted in the *upper left*. It converts alternating current from a wall source (50–60 Hz), to a radiofrequency output, typically about 500 KHz (500,000 Hz). The circuit is formed using two outlets. The three commercial examples shown each have similar colors for waveforms used for monopolar instrumentation—a low-voltage ("cut") output coded in *yellow* and a modulated high-voltage output ("coag") coded in *blue*. The "Force FX" (*upper right*) and the "System 5000" (*lower left*) each have a bipolar output that is coded in *blue*, even though the bipolar outputs are low voltage, similar to those of the *yellow-coded* "cut" outputs.

understand that the current in RF electrosurgery does not flow in one direction via the active and dispersive electrodes, but instead should be perceived as electrons (in the wires and ESU) or ions (in the tissue) rapidly oscillating back and forth.

All modern ESUs have ports for the two electrodes in the circuit, and controls that allow the surgeon to set the power output for each of the waveforms. While most North American-made ESUs have two outputs labeled *cut* and *coagulation* (or "coag"), these terms do not accurately reflect the appropriate use of the energy, a feature that tends to add to confusion regarding the properties and purpose of the different waveforms.

The output labeled "*cut*," when set at "pure," provides a continuous and relatively low-voltage waveform. As it is seen on the oscilloscope (Fig. 2.8a), the ESU output is in the form of a sine wave, reflecting both the continuous output from the generator, and the rapidly switching polarity of the AC.

a   Waveform - Low voltage, continuous

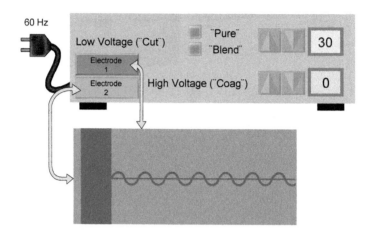

b Waveform - High voltage, modulated, dampened

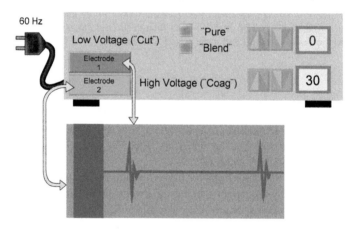

Fig. 2.8. The two basic waveforms are shown. (**a**) The image shows a low-voltage, continuous output in the form of a sine wave that is unfortunately called "cut" in North America, giving the false impression that it uniquely is designed for cutting tissue. (**b**) This panel shows a modulated (low duty cycle, typically about 6%), dampened, and high-voltage waveform that is also mischaracterized with the name "coag" in North American systems.

The so-called *"coagulation"* waveform is an interrupted, dampened, and relatively high-voltage waveform (Fig. 2.8b). Typically, the current is "on" only 6% of the time, referred to as a 6% *duty cycle*, and further described below.

Originally, *blended* outputs were created by combining the waveforms of two physically separate generators that produced the continuous low-voltage and modulated high-voltage waveforms described above. However, all modern ESUs create their "blended" outputs by producing interrupted (or modulated) versions of the continuous or pure "cut" waveforms. The term *duty cycle* is used to describe the percentage of time that the ESU is producing a waveform—if it is 80% of the time, it is referred to as an 80% duty cycle (Fig. 2.9a, b). When the current is interrupted, and therefore reduced, while the wattage is held constant, the generator increases the voltage of the output ($W = V \times I$). Alternatively stated, as the duty cycle diminishes, the voltage rises provided wattage is constant. In the water tower analogy, use of a "Blend" output is equivalent to slightly elevating the level of the tower while intermittently turning the water flow on and off at the tap. The flow of the water will pulse, and it will flow with a slightly higher pressure. Typically it is possible for the operator to vary the tissue effect by selecting from one or a number of blend modes that vary the duty cycle from, for example, 80–50%. This explanation also should facilitate understanding of the "coag" output, its low duty cycle, and relatively high voltage when set at the same power output on the ESU.

It is important to realize that all ESUs are not created equal. The duty cycles of the various "blend" modes vary from machine to machine. The peak voltages generated in any of the modes may vary significantly, depending, in part on the purpose for which the machine was designed. For example, machines designed for operating room use generally provide peak voltages for the continuous and blended outputs significantly higher than machines designed for office use.

Most ESUs designed for operating room use are capable of supporting bipolar instruments. This means that the dual wire bipolar cords attached to the bipolar instrument plug into the ESU and that there is a power output control specifically for the bipolar instrument (Fig. 2.7). Most modern generators provide only a continuous waveform from the bipolar outlets that is identical to the "cut" waveform. The reasons for this will be explained in subsequent sections.

There are a number of different ESU's on the market that are designed to support proprietary bipolar instruments such as Ligasure® (Covidien),

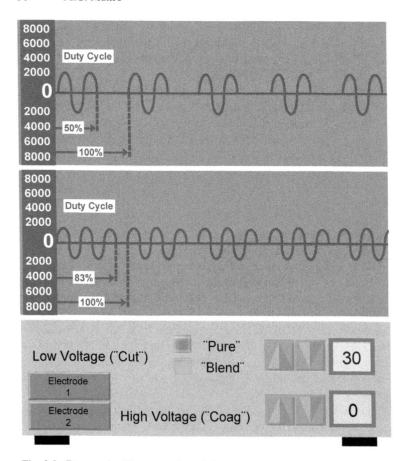

Fig. 2.9. Duty cycle. The proportion of time that the ESU is actually producing current is termed the "duty cycle." "Blended" currents are actually modulated low-voltage waveforms, NOT combinations of the "coag" and "cut" waveforms. On the *top panel*, there is output 50% of the time, whereas in the *middle panel*, it is 83% of the time. Note that to preserve the power equation ($P = V \times I$), with the decrease in current, there is a proportional increase in voltage with the lower duty cycle waveform.

PlasmaKinetics® (Olympus-Gyrus), and EnSeal® (Ethicon Endosurgery) (Fig. 2.10). These generators are designed with microprocessors that work with the bipolar device to measure impedance or temperature and vary features of the output such as voltage to customize the coagulation effects on the target tissue.

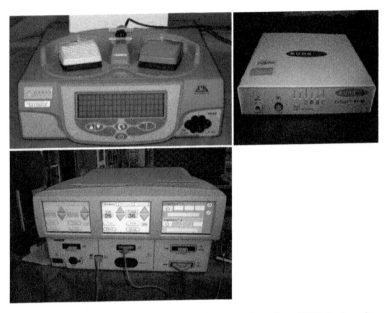

Fig. 2.10. Proprietary electrosurgical units. Depicted are three ESUs designed to run proprietary bipolar systems: The PlasmaKinetic system (Olympus-Gyrus, Inc.), *upper left*; the EnSeal system (Ethicon Endosurgery, Inc.), *upper right*; and the Force Triad that supports the LigaSure system (Covidien, Inc.), *lower left*. There are a number of different ESU's on the market that are designed to support proprietary bipolar instruments.

The Circuit: The System

Performance of electrosurgery requires the formation of an electrical circuit that includes the ESU, the electrodes and connecting wires, and, of course, the patient. The original systems were *ground referenced* meaning that the "ground" was an inherent part of the circuit, but all contemporary electrosurgical systems use isolated circuits, which means that the "ground" is excluded (Fig. 2.11).

At the risk of redundancy, a fundamental concept to have in mind when considering the circuits created for RF electrosurgery is that in each instance there must be two electrodes. Consequently *all RF electrosurgery is bipolar*. Whereas all systems have at least one of the electrodes designed to concentrate current sufficient to elevate local tissue and cause a surgical effect—what differentiates the systems is the location and purpose of the second electrode. This concept should also

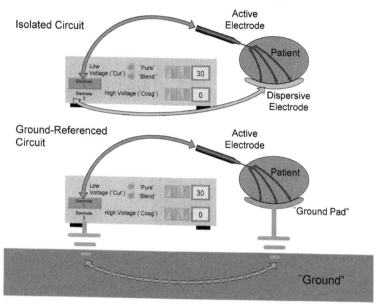

Fig. 2.11. Isolated vs. ground-references systems. Contemporary systems sold for operating room use are all designed with isolated circuits. Ground references systems depend on the "ground" to complete the circuit, a circumstance which brings into play the opportunity for current diversion through any potential circuit including EKG electrodes, and stirrups or other components of an operating room table.

include the notion that the part of the patient involved in the circuit is different between systems. For systems that use monopolar instruments the entire patient is involved, whereas in those systems that are designed for use with bipolar instruments, it is only the tissue interposed between the two electrodes that is involved in the circuit. These fundamental differences are responsible for a number of safety and performance differences between these systems (Fig. 2.4).

Monopolar Instruments and Systems

Monopolar systems include two separate monopolar instruments in the circuit, *the active electrode* and the *dispersive electrode*, between which is interposed the entire patient (Fig. 2.4). The active electrode is designed to focus the current or power on the surgical target thereby creating the desired tissue effect. The dispersive electrode is positioned on the patient in a location remote from the surgical site and is relatively large in surface area, a design that serves to defocus or disperse the current thereby preventing tissue injury.

Active electrodes can have many designs, but those with a point, hook, narrow tip, or bladed edge are generally used to concentrate current and power, for the purpose of tissue vaporization and cutting (Fig. 2.12). When the active electrode has a slightly larger surface area, such as the side of a blade or when it is shaped like a ball or is in the form of a grasper, the same output used for cutting will result only in local coagulation and desiccation, and, consequently, can be used for the purpose of hemostasis. A better name for the active electrode might be

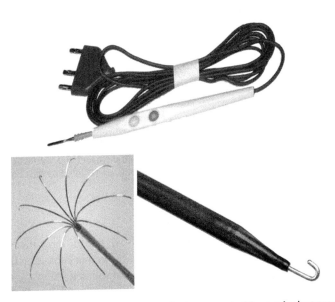

Fig. 2.12. "Active" electrodes in monopolar instruments. Monopolar instruments comprise only one electrode. The *top* is a hand-held electrode for open surgery. Note that there are three prongs on the plug—only one is necessary, but some systems are designed to include monitoring systems (for impedance for example). *Lower right* is a laparoscopic monopolar instrument with a hook electrode and an insulated shaft. In the *lower left* is a multitined monopolar electrode in a monopolar instrument designed for ablation of large volumes of tissue—so-called radiofrequency ablation (see Chap. 9).

34   M.G. Munro

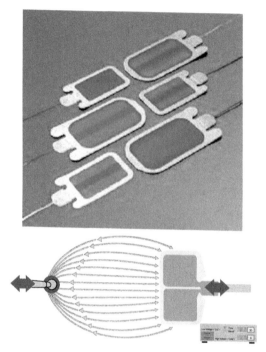

Fig. 2.13. Dispersive electrodes. Several dispersive electrodes are shown (*top*). Note that some actually comprise two separate electrodes, the so-called "split pad" that allows for the detection of a partial detachment if the ESU is capable of measuring and comparing the impedance in each electrode. Note the diagram below demonstrating the bidirectional nature of the current and the fact that the same current is focused by the active electrode (*left*) and diluted by the dispersive electrode (*right*).

the "power or current concentrating electrode," but for most this would be a mouthful so we will use "active electrode" in this book even though dispersive electrodes can become "active" as discussed below.

Dispersive electrodes are almost always designed with an adhesive to facilitate continuing contact with the patient and prevention of a clinically significant local thermal effect (Fig. 2.13). However, if there is partial detachment, the current or power density will increase, and the dispersive electrode can become "active" and capable of creating thermal injury, often called a "burn." Most (but not all) ESUs sold in the past 20 years are designed to measure the impedance at the level of the dispersive electrode, a function that also requires specialized dispersive electrode design. Usually this is in the form of a "split pad" which, effectively, is two dispersive electrodes in one (Fig. 2.13). A difference in the measured impedance in the two dispersive electrodes will generally reflect partial attachment (or detachment) and the machine will not start, or, if already "on," will shut off automatically.

Hopefully this description will help the reader understand the reason that the terms "return" and "ground," when used to describe the electrode designed to disperse current, are both inaccurate and confusing. The continuously switching polarity of ACs means that there is no net electron flow. Consequently, neither electrode should be perceived as being dedicated to "return" current or electrons to the ESU. Virtually, all ESUs designed for the operating room and sold in the last 30 or more years have isolated circuits, and there is no reference to "ground" in the system.

Bipolar Instruments and Systems

Simply put, bipolar systems are designed to use instruments designed with both electrodes positioned on the same surgical device (Fig. 2.14). Consequently, instead of a single wire connecting the ESU and the dispersive electrode and another linking the ESU to the "active" electrode, both are contained in one cable that joins the generator to the bipolar instrument. A fundamental concept is that the only part of the patient involved in the circuit is the tissue interposed between the two electrodes, a design that prevents complications related to current diversion and provides more accurate measurements of local tissue parameters such as temperature and impedance. However, bipolar systems also have limitations, as it is more difficult to include a method for electrosurgical vaporization and cutting into the design.

The simplest bipolar instruments contain two flat monopolar electrodes, electrically isolated from each other in the device. The electrodes are generally flat and in some fashion articulated, a design that allows the surgeon to grasp and compress tissue. With this configuration, both electrodes are "active" in that they are equally capable of elevating as the local temperature sufficiently to cause the processes of coagulation and desiccation discussed below. Most of the proprietary systems are based on this concept but include a sliding mechanical knife if they are designed to both coagulate and cut tissue. In addition, these proprietary

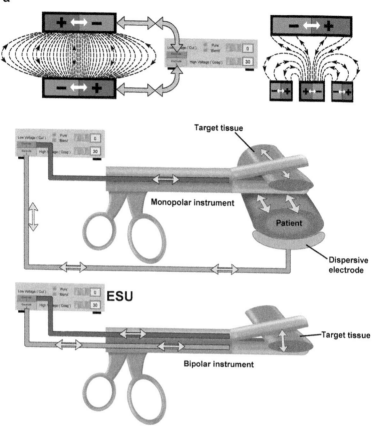

Fig. 2.14. Bipolar versus monopolar instruments. The two electrodes in a bipolar instrument constantly change polarity, at a rate determined by the generator, generally about 500 MHz. ((a), *top left*). Some bipolar instruments have a more complicated design or arrangement of the two electrodes. In the example ((a), *top right*), the *upper* and *lower left* and *right* components are really one "electrode" while the second electrode is in the *middle* of the *bottom row*, an arrangement that can result in cutting activity because the lower middle component creates a high current density. The lower figures in (a) show that two instruments that may seem similar in design are actually quite different, the *top* instrument is monopolar as the jaws of the grasper are joined creating a single electrode. Note that there is a dispersive electrode that the entire patient is involved in the circuit, and that there is one wire into the instrument. The *bottom* instrument is actually bipolar—the two wires entering the instrument from the generator each connect to one of the jaws that are insulated from each other. Only the tissue between the jaws becomes part of the circuit. (b) These differences are demonstrated with real instruments, a monopolar grasper (A) and a bipolar grasper (B). Note in the *lower right panel* that there is an insulator between the jaws in (B) that is not present in (A). In the *lower left panel*, the single electrosurgical "post" of a monopolar instrument is shown, while the double wire and multiple prongs for the bipolar instrument are shown in (B).

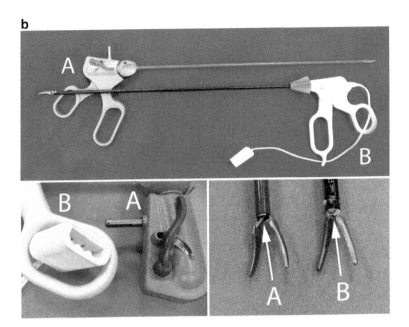

Fig. 2.14. (continued)

systems measure local tissue impedance and/or temperature in an attempt to more accurately define an "end point" for vessel sealing, based on the knowledge that certain temperature thresholds or high impedance levels are associated with complete tissue coagulation and desiccation. The details of these systems are discussed in a later chapter.

While it is difficult to design bipolar instruments for cutting, it is possible, and there are a number of such systems currently marketed. One approach is to design the instrument so that when placed on tissue an electrode with a relatively large surface area is in contact with tissue, while simultaneously a narrow blade or needle electrode is used to cut. Another is a design that joins both "grasping" components into one electrode, while a blade that is positioned along the tissue serves as the active electrode. A bipolar needle electrode is shown in (Fig. 2.15).

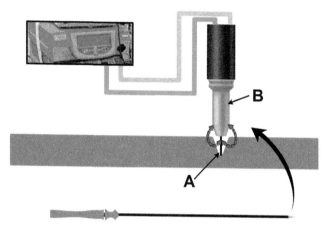

Fig. 2.15. Bipolar cutting instrument. This graphic depicts another bipolar instrument designed for cutting. The needle electrode (**A**) is isolated from the larger and proximal dispersive electrode (**B**). The instrument is connected to the proprietary ESU by a dedicated cable. The *red dotted lines* pathway demonstrates the current pathway between the two electrodes; the zone of vaporization is depicted around the needle electrode.

Effect of Temperature on Cells and Tissue

Understanding the surgical applications of RF electricity requires a basic understanding of the effects of temperature on cells and tissue (Fig. 2.16). Normal body temperature is 37°C and all of us, from time to time, when we have infections, experience temperature elevations that can reach as high as 40°C or so without damage to the structural integrity of our cells and tissue. However, when cellular temperature reaches 50°C cell death will occur in approximately 6 min [16] and if the local temperature is 60°C cellular death is instantaneous [17].

So what happens at 60°C? Between about 60 and 95°C (in effect, below 100 degrees C) two simultaneous processes occur that are of interest to surgeons. The first is protein denaturation that occurs secondary to the impact of temperature on the hydrothermal bonds that exist between protein molecules. When the local temperature is as low as 60°C, these bonds are instantaneously broken but then quickly reform, as the local temperature cools. This ideally leads to a homogenous coagulum, a process that is typically called "coagulation." The other

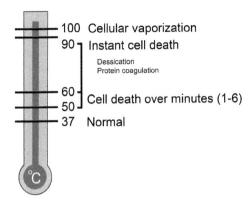

Fig. 2.16. Impact of temperature on cells and tissue. Normal body temperature is 37°C, and if cellular or tissue temperature reaches 50°C for 6 min, cell death occurs. If the temperature reaches 60°C, cell death occurs instantaneously. If the temperature is less than 100°C, but at least 60°C, the mechanisms involved in cell death include cellular desiccation and protein coagulation. When the intracellular temperature reaches 100°C, cellular vaporization occurs secondary to a liquid–gas conversion to steam.

effect is dehydration or *desiccation* as the cells lose water through the thermally damaged cellular wall. From a gross and microscopic perspective, so-called *white coagulation* is the result of a process similar to boiling the white of an egg—a white, homogenous coagulum. Microscopically it has been demonstrated that protein bonds are formed creating the homogenous, gelatinous structure. Such a tissue effect is useful for occluding tubular structures such as fallopian tubes, or blood vessels for the purpose of hemostasis.

If the intracellular temperature rises to 100°C or more, a liquid–gaseous conversion occurs as the intracellular water boils forming steam. The subsequent massive intracellular expansion results in explosive vaporization of the cell with a cloud of steam, ions, and organic matter. It is suspected that the explosive force results in acoustical vibrations that contribute to the cutting effect through the tissue.

When the local temperature reaches higher levels, such as temperature reaches 200°C or more, the organic molecules are broken down in a process called *carbonization*. This leaves the carbon molecules that create a black and/or brown appearance, sometimes referred to as "black coagulation."

Effect of Alternating Current on Cells

The process called electrosurgery is based on the ability of the RF current to elevate cellular, and, consequently, tissue temperature to attain the desired tissue effect. Understanding how this occurs starts with the knowledge of the impact of RF electromagnetic energy on intracellular components.

There are at least two basic mechanisms whereby RF electricity increases cellular and tissue temperature. The most important is by the conversion of electromagnetic energy to mechanical energy, which then is converted to thermal energy by frictional forces. A second, and likely less important mechanism, is resistive heating, where current flowing across a resistor causes an increase in the temperature of that resistor. These mechanisms will be discussed below. A third and indirect mechanism of tissue heating is conductive heat transfer, the tissue adjacent to that which undergoes the direct effects of RF electricity.

Conversion of Radiofrequency Electromagnetic Energy to Mechanical Energy

Cellular cytoplasm contains electrically charged particles or ions in the form of atoms and molecules (Fig. 2.17). Cations are small, positively charged atoms like sodium, potassium, and calcium, while the anions include atoms such as chlorine as well as large, negatively charged protein molecules. If a DC, with its constant polarity, is applied to the cell, the cations tend to migrate toward the direction of the negative electrode while the anions orient to the positive electrode as unidirectional current flow is established (Fig. 2.17, top panel). This is called the *galvanic effect*, and has no known medical purpose.

When an AC, with its continuously switching polarity, is applied to the cell, the anions and cations migrate to the positive and negative poles respectively, but, rather than maintaining an orientation within the cell, they oscillate in synchrony with the changing polarity of the output (Fig. 2.17, bottom panel).

If the frequency of the AC is relatively low (20–30 kHz), the impact of the RF energy will incite depolarization of muscles and nerves and the creation of action potentials that result in muscle fasciculation and related pain, a process known as the *Faradic Effect*. It is thought that this

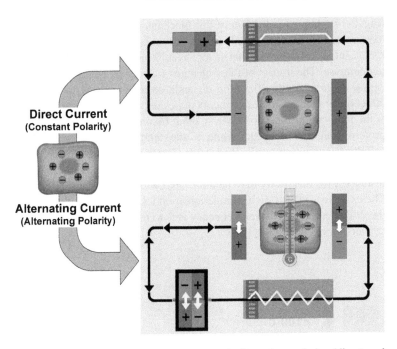

Fig. 2.17. Cellular response to constant and alternating polarity (direct and alternating current). Cells contain anions (negatively charged) and cations (positively charged). When a direct current is applied to a cell (*top right panel*), the anions tend to migrate within the cytoplasm toward the positive pole and the cations to the negative pole. However, when the polarity changes 500,000 times per second, the electromagnetic energy is converted to mechanical energy as the molecules rapidly oscillate within the cytoplasm (*bottom right panel*). With this rapid motion and, especially in the instance of large protein molecules, frictional forces result in the conversion of the mechanical energy to thermal energy.

depolarization is initiated through voltage-gated sodium and/or calcium ion channels that exist within neural and muscular cell membranes. However, nerve and muscle membranes are not sensitive to the very short duration "pulses" characteristic of the high-frequency electromagnetic energy in the RF spectrum. Consequently, when RF (100 kHz–3.0 MHz), AC is applied across the cell, the pulse duration is so short that the sodium and calcium ionic channel gates do not open, and cellular membrane depolarization doesn't occur. Instead, the electromagnetic energy is converted into mechanical energy as the cations and anions rapidly oscillate within the cellular cytoplasm

(Fig. 2.17). Almost immediately, this mechanical energy, and especially that created by the large oscillating proteins, is converted, by frictional forces, into thermal energy that, in turn, results in elevation of intracellular temperature. The impact of these changes was discussed above, and the degree of temperature elevation depends on a number of factors that affect the amount of Joules of energy deposited in a given tissue volume. If the temperature rises to between about 60 and 95°C, desiccation and protein coagulation occur, while if the temperature reaches 100°C cellular vaporization results (Fig. 2.18). The factors involved in creating these different surgical effects are discussed in the next section. In some instances, RF electricity may be associated with muscle depolarization. The exact reasons for such stimulation are not known, but could include the influence of stray lower frequency arcs to tissue, or rectification, the conversion of AC to DC [18].

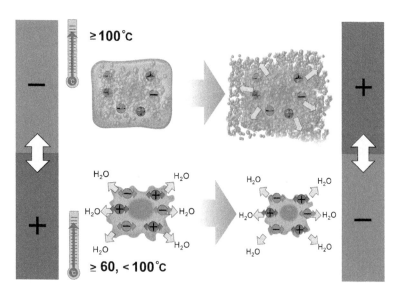

Fig. 2.18. Impact of elevated temperature on cells. If enough energy is transmitted to the cell sufficient to increase the temperature to at least 60°C, but below 100°C, there is loss of cellular water (desiccation) through the damaged cell wall (*bottom*). On the other hand, if the temperature meets or exceeds 100°C (*top*), the intracellular water turns to steam, there is massive expansion of the intracellular volume, and the cell explodes in a cloud of steam, ions, and organic matter—the process of vaporization.

Resistive Heating

When either AC or DC flows through a resistor, the resulting effect is the generation of heat, much like the response of a filament in a light bulb. Alternately stated, the resistance of the tissue converts the electric energy of the voltage source into thermal energy that causes the tissue temperature to rise. This relationship is defined in *Joules Laws* after the nineteenth century English physicist James Precott Joule (Table 2.2). It is likely that this mechanism comes into play after the primary mechanism of ionic oscillation described above results in increased tissue impedance by virtue of cellular dehydration or desiccation. In the process of fulguration, superficial coagulation is achieved very quickly, but subsequently tissue temperature rises to levels not seen with typical cutting or "white" coagulation. Consequently, it is likely that the very high temperatures reached are secondary to resistive heating.

Tissue Effects of Electrosurgery

The concepts around creation of a given tissue effect using RF electricity are extensions of the impact of the energy on cells. The tissue effects depend upon a number of factors including the power output of the ESU, the waveform of the output, the impedance of the target tissue, the area of the electrode interfacing with the tissue, and the proximity of the electrode to the target tissue (contact or noncontact). Another factor is the distension medium utilized for the procedure. The basic principles will be discussed under the appropriate headings; then will follow a discussion of the factors that modify the tissue effect.

Cutting

Formation of a tissue incision with RF electricity is simply the process of linear vaporization. Vaporization of tissue is best achieved with a continuous, low-voltage waveform, using a unipolar instrument with a narrow, pointed or blade-shaped electrode held near to but not in contact with the tissue. The generator is activated, allowing the thin electrode to concentrate the current and therefore the power at its tip—a high power density. The current then arcs between the electrode and the tissue, rapidly elevating the local intracellular temperature to more than 100°C causing

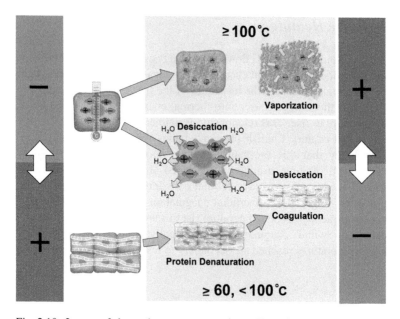

Fig. 2.19. Impact of elevated temperature on tissue. To understand the formation of an electrosurgically-induced vessel seal, it is important to understand the tissue impact of elevation of tissue temperature at least 60°C, but below 100°C. The first is tissue desiccation, which is just the tissue manifestation of mass cellular dehydration and resulting volumetric shrinkage. The second is the rupture of hydrothermal bonds or crosslinks and reformation of these in a random fashion that includes bridging the gap between two opposing tissue surfaces. Provided these tissues are somewhat similar in protein content, the result will be a strong seal, as if the vessel walls were compressed and welded together. Cutting or transection of tissue electrosurgically requires the establishment of a localized zone of vaporization followed by linear extension of this zone keeping the electrode within the vapor or steam "pocket" or "envelope" created by the vaporized tissue.

focused cellular vaporization and the creation of a local "plasma cloud" of steam, ions, and organic matter. To extend this zone of vaporization and form an incision, the electrode is advanced, keeping its tip or edge and the target tissue within the plasma cloud or "steam envelope" (Fig. 2.19). Because the voltage is low and the current dissipates rapidly with distance from the active electrode, the thermal damage on each side of the cut zone is minimal, provided the use of both appropriate equipment and surgical technique.

The actual depth and extent of adjacent coagulation injury incurred in association with an electrosurgically created incision is dependent upon a

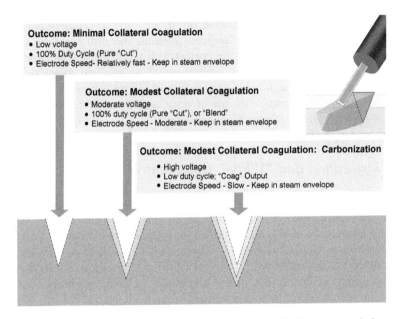

Outcome: Minimal Collateral Coagulation
- Low voltage
- 100% Duty Cycle (Pure "Cut")
- Electrode Speed- Relatively fast - Keep in steam envelope

Outcome: Modest Collateral Coagulation
- Moderate voltage
- 100% duty cycle (Pure "Cut"), or "Blend"
- Electrode Speed - Moderate - Keep in steam envelope

Outcome: Modest Collateral Coagulation: Carbonization
- High voltage
- Low duty cycle; "Coag" Output
- Electrode Speed - Slow - Keep in steam envelope

Fig. 2.20. Factors affecting depth and characteristics of adjacent coagulation when cutting tissue using RF electrosurgery. The major characteristics are the voltage, the waveform, and the electrode speed. In general, the slower the speed, the more energy delivered to adjacent tissue. However, if the speed of the electrode is too fast, it will get ahead of the steam envelope, a circumstance that results in contact with the tissue, transiently lower current density, and the creation of a zone of desiccation and coagulation. Higher voltage can be created by using a lower duty cycle, or turning up the generator (or both). The result is more adjacent coagulation injury. If a modulated high-voltage ("coag") waveform is used, everything else being equal, there will be more collateral coagulation and carbonization as very high local temperatures can be reached.

number of factors including power output, electrode size and shape, waveform and peak voltage, and the speed and skill of the surgeon. Consequently, descriptions of the depth of coagulation injury should take the existence of such variables into consideration (Fig. 2.20). While the minimum depth of thermal injury has been described as low as a few microns [19], more typical reported peritoneal injury studies suggest depth of thermal injury from less than 200 μm for pure cutting waveforms [20] to 300 μm for blended waveforms [21]. Such injury depths no doubt, reflect, in part, the rather high peak voltage outputs of the generators currently in general use.

While bipolar cutting instruments exist, they are difficult to design because of the requirement for the two electrodes to be oriented in a way that allows efficient vaporization to occur. Bipolar needle-tipped instruments require that the surgeon maintain the instrument in an orientation that maintains tissue contact with the dispersive electrode (Fig. 2.15). Some innovative electrosurgical sealing and transection instruments that use bipolar cutting techniques have been designed. These instruments require the use of waveforms designed to overcome the high impedance of the coagulated tissue.

Desiccation and "White" Coagulation

As described previously, two simultaneous processes occur when tissue temperature is maintained at 50°C for at least 6 min, or instantaneously at 60–95°C—protein coagulation and dehydration or desiccation. Unlike the case for vaporization, the cellular proteins are altered but not destroyed. While two distinct intracellular effects are occurring simultaneously, many use either the term coagulation or desiccation to describe both processes.

Effective coagulation for the purposes of sealing vessels or other lumen-containing structures requires contact of the electrode with tissue. When a blunt or flat electrode is placed in contact with the tissue, all the energy on that electrode is made available for conversion to intracellular heat by the processes described previously in this section. In conjunction with properly selected power outputs, the power density is high enough to cause instantaneous coagulation and desiccation, but not so high as to elevate the intracellular temperature to 100°C where vaporization would occur (Fig. 2.21).

Although any waveform may be used to create tissue coagulation and desiccation, a continuous low-voltage output ("cut") results in a predictable zone of coagulation with higher quality and consistency than that achieved with the output labeled "coagulation." There are a number of reasons for this apparent paradox. First, compared to low-voltage waveforms, the modulated "coagulation" waveform results in an uneven amount of protein bonding, limiting the ability to, for example, achieve complete occlusion of a blood vessel (Fig. 2.22). In addition, such waveforms cause the more superficial layers of the tissue to become rapidly coagulated, increasing impedance, thereby preventing further transmission of the energy to the deeper layers of the tissue [22]. Finally, the temperature generated near the electrode may exceed 200°C, causing carbonization and breakdown of molecules to sugars, a process that

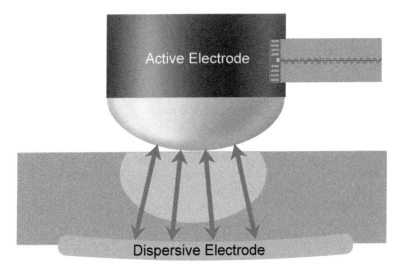

Fig. 2.21. Coagulation with low-voltage continuous waveform ("cut"). The process of tissue coagulation is best achieved using a continuous low-voltage output.

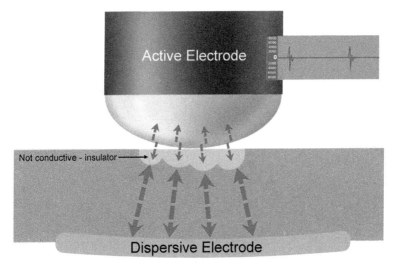

Fig. 2.22. Coagulation with modulated high-voltage waveform ("coag"). This figure demonstrates the impact of modulated high-voltage waveforms on tissue when coagulation is attempted. The intermittent output from the 6% duty cycle waveform causes a brief and superficial elevation of tissue temperature, sufficient to cause focal coagulation, desiccation, and, in many instances, carbonization. The next time a burst or arc returns to this area, the tissue impedance has risen sharply, so the current is blocked or diverts to a less impedant zone of tissue. This approach creates a superficial and inhomogeneous zone of desiccation and coagulation, not suitable for vessel sealing.

facilitates adherence of the electrode to tissue, allowing the eschar to be pulled off with removal of the electrode, a process that can disrupt the already suboptimal vessel seal and cause bleeding.

As a result of these considerations, coagulation should be performed with monopolar or bipolar instruments containing electrodes that have a relatively large surface area, and using the continuous and relatively low-voltage "cutting" waveform. If a blood vessel is to be coagulated, it should be first coapted by compressing it against adjacent tissue or, preferably, by grasping it with a forceps (Fig. 2.23). These maneuvers facilitate the formation of a vascular seal by preventing the flow of blood from removing heat from the site, and juxtapose the vessel walls, thereby allowing the vascular seal to be created.

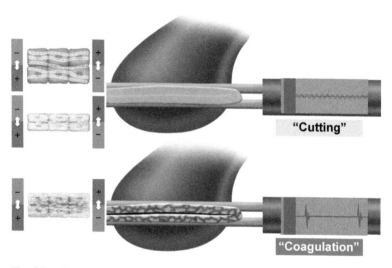

Fig. 2.23. Use low voltage ("cut") to seal vessels. This figure demonstrates the difference between using low-voltage continuous outputs, and modulated high-voltage outputs when trying to seal a vessel. The low-voltage output (*top*) results in a homogenous vessel seal. The modulated high-voltage output (*bottom*) creates a superficial and inhomogeneous zone of desiccation and coagulation as well as carbonization and caramelization as proteins are reduced to sugars. This combination creates a poor vessel seal, and facilitates sticking of the tissue to the forceps, a process that facilitates disruption of the seal with forceps removal.

Fulguration

Fulguration is a process whereby the tissue is superficially coagulated by repeated high-voltage electrosurgical arcs that continue to elevate the temperature by resistive heating to beyond 100°, reaching levels of 200°C and more. In addition to coagulation and desiccation, there is breakdown of the organic molecules into their atomic components including carbon that results in the addition of a dark hue to the coagulated tissue that is called "carbonization." This process probably requires local temperatures of 400°C or more has also been described as *spray coagulation* or *black coagulation* (Fig. 2.24).

The process of arcing the current between the electrode and tissue is accomplished using the modulated high-voltage waveform labeled "coagulation" on most North American ESUs. Remember that this waveform has a very low duty cycle (typically 6%) but very high voltage that effectively manifests as pulses of high voltage current. The active electrode is held a few millimeters away from the tissue at a distance sufficient to allow ionization of the media in the electrode–tissue gap with subsequent establishment of visible arcs between the two structures

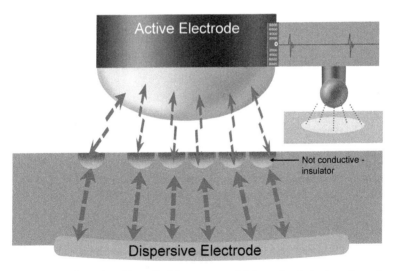

Fig. 2.24. Fulguration ("coag"). The process of fulguration is best performed with the high-voltage modulated outputs called "coag" on most ESUs. It is best to hold the electrode near to but not in contact with tissue. Care should be exercised as this arrangement can create an "open circuit" situation that can facilitate capacitive coupling.

(electrode and tissue). Unlike the case of low-voltage continuous current, the interrupted high-voltage discharges identify variable paths to the tissue and manifest in what appears to be a spraying effect onto an area of tissue that is much larger than the electrode itself. When a current pulse impacts a focal area of tissue, intracellular temperatures increase, but then reduce again because of the lack of sustained current in that focal area. The result is a relatively diffuse, inhomogeneous zone of elevated tissue temperature causing coagulation and carbonization that is limited to the superficial tissue layers, typically to a depth of about 0.5 mm. The rapid, superficial nature of this type of coagulation raises tissue impedance, inhibiting propagation of the thermal effect by preventing the current from including the deeper layers of the tissue. Consequently, this type of coagulation is most preferred for the arrest of capillary or small arteriolar bleeding over a large surface area.

Variables Impacting the Tissue Effects of Electrosurgery

After the basic principles of electrosurgery are understood, the next step is to learn how to modify the tissue effects by changing one or more aspects of technique. Familiarity with these variables is essential for safe and effective application of RF electricity.

Power Density

The power density is the total wattage striking the tissue per unit area of the electrode adjacent to or in contact with that tissue. This variable is of paramount importance in the performance of electrosurgery. Power density is determined by a combination of the shape and size of the electrode and the power settings and output of the ESU.

Electrode Surface Area

As discussed previously, the power density required to vaporize tissue must be very high, which in turn requires the use of an electrode with a very small surface area. Some electrodes may be designed to serve a dual purpose. For example, a blade-shaped electrode may be employed as a cutting device if the blade's narrow edge is held near to the tissue, creating a zone of high power density. Alternatively, by placing the breadth of the blade in contact with the tissue, the resultant

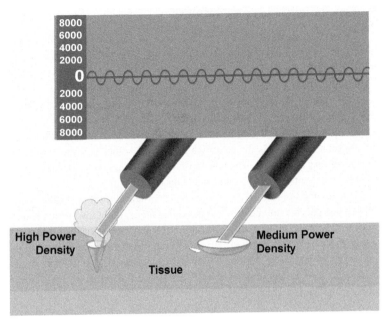

Fig. 2.25. Changing current/power density with a blade electrode. A blade electrode demonstrates that it is the current/power density, not the waveform, that is responsible for the difference between vaporization and coagulation. Using the same low-voltage output, the edge of the blade (*left*) focuses the current/power on the tissue while at the same output, the side of the blade defocuses the current/power. The result is vaporization/cutting with the blade edge and tissue desiccation/coagulation with the side of the blade.

lower power density can be used for coagulation (Fig. 2.25). Note that if the leading edge of the blade is used for cutting purposes, the flat sides may contact the edge of the incision as the electrode is passed through tissue, creating an additional degree of adjacent tissue coagulation. Depending upon the clinical situation, this effect may be either an advantage or disadvantage.

As discussed previously, the electrode at the other end of the power density spectrum is the *dispersive electrode*. Given the same power output and waveform, such electrodes properly attached to the patient dissipate the current so much that there is no thermal effect on cells and tissue.

Fulgurating electrodes are preferably similar to those designed for coagulation, or can be shaped in the form of a ball. This reduces the power density, and facilitates the spraying effect created by the high-voltage output.

Electrosurgical Generator Power Output

An understanding of the output characteristics of the ESU will enable the surgeon more effectively to vary the power density. It is important to know that different generator brands have different output characteristics with varying peak voltages and variable duty cycles at the blend settings. These variables will, in many instances, affect subtleties of technique and the effect on tissue. Virtually all ESUs have a means by which the output in watts may be controlled or set. Contemporary ESUs have an LED screen that reveals the exact wattage, while older systems that may still be in use have a logarithmic scale from 1 (lowest) to 10 (highest), making exact settings and adjustments more difficult.

As discussed previously in this chapter, power output is proportional to both the voltage and current. In most instances, the appropriate power output for cutting will be the minimum amount necessary to create the power density at the electrode tip that results in desired combination of vaporization and coagulation. When using RF electricity to fashion an incision, more power means more voltage and increased coagulation adjacent to the cut area.

The voltage may be incrementally increased without changing the power settings by using *"blended waveforms"* with their increased peak voltage. Such waveforms result in greater thermal injury around an incision because the higher voltage pushes more joules of energy into tissue and the interrupted nature of the current dictates a slower cutting speed. This effect may be exploited when hemostasis is necessary along an incision line or when transecting tissue that has relatively high impedance.

Tissue Impedance or Resistance

Whereas each component of an electrical circuit contributes to impedance, tissue impedance is the one most important to the surgeon. Highly conductive tissues have a high water content and offer little resistance to the passage of current and the creation of a desired tissue effect. However, it is the tissue itself that provides the greatest degree of variability. Tissue that offers high impedance is generally low in fluid content and therefore relatively nonconductive. Tissue such as bone, calloused skin, fat, or any previously desiccated tissue will impede passage of current and therefore will inhibit the creation of an electrosurgical effect.

If it is necessary to cut through tissue with relatively high impedance, increasing the voltage by raising the power output or decreasing the duty cycle is usually effective. In such cases, the current is pushed through the relatively resistant tissue with greater force.

Waveform

The impact of RF energy on tissue effect is also related to the waveform of the output of the ESU. Throughout this chapter we have emphasized the fact that the labels of the settings on the ESU are frequently misleading (e.g., "cut," "coagulation"), so an understanding of the underlying rationale is important. In addition, it should be emphasized that the "coagulation" output by virtue of its much higher voltage (typically 3x compared to "cutting" for a given wattage) is associated with higher risks of instrument insulation breakdown and current diversion. Consequently, in the few instances where such outputs are necessary, increased care should be taken to protect adjacent and surrounding tissue.

High Voltage, Modulated, and Dampened ("Coagulation")

The principle use of this modulated high-voltage waveform is for the process of *fulguration*. Some contemporary generators have a number of additional selections or controls that are labeled in a number of ways, such as "fulgurate" or "spray." In general, "spray" has the lowest duty cycle and the highest peak voltage. As will be discussed in later chapters, and especially during laparoscopy, use of these high voltages should be selective and the operator should understand the increased risks of insulation damage and capacitive coupling.

There are circumstances when high-voltage waveforms may be useful or necessary for efficient cutting. One such instance occurs when it is necessary to transect high impedance surgical targets such as fat, scars, and tissue that are previously desiccated. In such circumstances, the surgeon can increase the wattage output on the ESU or an output of similar wattage can be selected with higher voltage such as the "blend" settings or the highly modulated "coagulation" output. Indeed, the waveform used for inert gas enhanced electrosurgery (e.g., Argon Beam Coagulator®) is a modulated high-voltage output.

Low-Voltage Continuous or Modulated ("Cutting")

The low-voltage continuous outputs are generally the most efficient and effective for either cutting (linear vaporization) or for coagulation/desiccation, including sealing blood vessels.

For tissue transection, the continuous low-voltage outputs ("cut") are generally both effective and safe. As previously stated, higher-voltage waveforms may be necessary when it is necessary to cut high impedance surgical targets such as fat, scars, and tissue that are previously desiccated. In such circumstances, the "blend" settings provide a slightly higher voltage and are an alternative to increasing the power output.

As described previously in this chapter, when the desired tissue effect is coagulation the generator output should be the low-voltage continuous output provided by the "cut" setting. Such waveforms, by virtue of their low voltage and continuous output, provide the most homogenous and deep coagulation and desiccation, and, therefore, are the best for creating a vascular seal. For proprietary bipolar systems, such outputs are intrinsically set—the surgeon has no control, and for the vast majority of generic ESUs, the bipolar outputs are also predetermined to have continuous low-voltage output (despite the "blue" color coding applied to most North American systems). However, when using unipolar instruments for coagulation, regardless of the approach (laparoscopic or laparotomic) the "yellow" low-voltage "cut" setting should be selected when sealing blood vessels.

Time on or Near Tissue

The amount of energy imparted to a given volume of tissue is directly related to the time the activated electrode is near to or in contact with that tissue, provided the voltage is low enough to prevent proximal coagulation, as discussed above. The circumstance is somewhat obvious for tissue coagulation, but it can impact the tissue effects of cutting as well. For example, if, when used for cutting, the electrode is moved very slowly through tissue, there will occur a greater degree of collateral thermal injury. However, moving the electrode too quickly will also result in increased thermal injury if the electrode moves ahead of the steam or vapor cloud and touches the tissue reducing the power density causing coagulation (Fig. 2.20).

Electrode–Tissue Relationships

An important factor in the performance of electrosurgery is the relationship of the active electrode to the target tissue. For the process of cutting, which we are portraying as linear vaporization, the relationship between the electrode and tissue could be described as *near-contact*. In this relationship, the current arcs between the active electrode and the tissue within the steam envelope generated by the vaporized intracellular contents. If the electrode is held too far from the tissue, no arcing and, therefore, no vaporization will occur. On the other hand, if the electrode touches the tissue, the power density decreases and coagulation will occur, creating a greater degree of thermal injury to the tissue adjacent to the incision line.

As previously described, fulguration is also a non- or near-contact electrosurgical activity facilitated by the use of the high-voltage, modulated waveform, usually with a short (e.g., 6%) duty cycle. Because of the higher voltage, the electrode can be held a millimeter or more from the target, while the current is "sprayed" onto the tissue. The distance that the electrode is held from the tissue is dependent in part upon the specific generator and the peak voltage in the "coagulation" setting.

For practical purposes, the processes of clinically effective white coagulation and desiccation are best achieved when there is contact between the electrode and the tissue. Implicitly, such electrodes have a flattened surface that facilitates creation of the required lower power density. In most instances, the instruments (both bipolar and monopolar) are designed as articulated grasping forceps that can compress the tissue between their jaws thereby coapting blood vessels to facilitate hemostatic sealing when activated, a process called coaptive coagulation.

Another important concept is compressed tissue volume. The larger the tissue thickness between the jaws of an RF electrosurgical instrument, regardless of its fundamental design (monopolar or bipolar), the greater the number of Joules of energy that will be required for complete coagulation and desiccation. What this means is that thicker pedicles will result in more lateral extension of the electrosurgical thermal injury, a factor that may be enhanced with monopolar instruments. Such an effect may have little clinical relevance in some situations, but, when operating near vital structures, injury could occur.

Media Between Electrode and Tissue

An often-forgotten component of the electrical circuit is the medium that exists between the electrode and the tissue, provided near-contact technique is used. The arc between electrode and tissue occurs only when the electrical field between the active electrode and the tissue becomes strong enough to ionize the intervening medium. These ions collide with other molecules until the charge crosses the gap between electrode and tissue, completing the circuit (Fig. 2.26).

Different media possess varying ionizing capabilities. For example, the CO_2 medium employed for most laparoscopy cases is only 70% as effective as room air at transmitting a charge. On the other hand, the

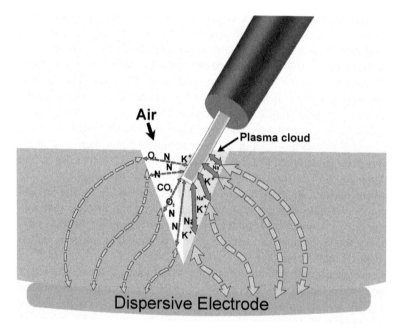

Fig. 2.26. Media and electrosurgery. The electrical properties of the media (air, CO_2, water, saline, etc.) around the active electrode are included in the electrical circuit, especially if the electrode is held off the tissue. Consequently, the impedance in a steam envelope or "plasma cloud" that includes sodium, potassium, and other ions (*right side above*), is much lower than that of air that is largely nitrogen and oxygen or especially carbon dioxide that comprises most laparoscopic environments. With monopolar systems, saline or blood around the electrode can make it function like a dispersive electrode, severely impeding performance.

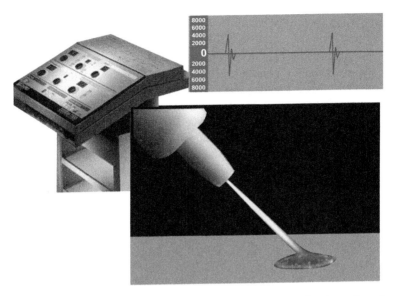

Fig. 2.27. Argon beam coagulator. Argon interposed between the electrode and the tissue is a medium that facilitates arcing of the current between the target and the active electrode. This is exploited in the argon beam coagulator and other similar systems that actually use a modulated low-voltage output to cut tissue at a distance from the electrode. The current ionizes the otherwise inert argon gas, creating a zone of low impedance through the air between the active electrode and the tissue.

plasma cloud that results from cellular vaporization contains large numbers of ions, a feature that makes it highly conductive. Argon gas also promotes conductivity of electrical current, a feature that is exploited by the Argon Beam Coagulator (Fig. 2.27), which is essentially an instrument that allows arcing of high-voltage outputs to occur from a distance of 1 to 2 cm.

Other Important Variables

There are other concepts important for the effective use of electrosurgery. For example, active electrodes must be kept shiny and free of carbon, as carbon deposits act as insulators impeding the flow of current. In addition, a moist electrode and tissue will facilitate the formation of the steam envelope necessary for effective vaporization and cutting, a characteristic exploited in electromicrosurgery.

Summary

RF electrosurgery used appropriately allows the surgeon to perform a wide spectrum of procedures safely, effectively, and with minimal undesired tissue trauma. Used without proper care, education, and training, electrosurgery, like other instruments and energy sources, has the potential to cause excessive tissue trauma, and increased operative morbidity, sometimes of a life-threatening nature. This chapter provides the reader with a fundamental knowledge of the scientific principles of RF electrosurgery that will facilitate understanding of the systems and techniques discussed elsewhere in this volume.

References

1. Cushing H, Bovie W. Electrosurgery as an aid to the removal of intracranial tumors. Surg Gynecol Obstet. 1928;47:751–84.
2. Major RH. History of medicine volumes I and II. Springfield: Charles C. Thomas; 1954.
3. Licht SH. The history of therapeutic heat. 2nd ed. New Haven: Elizabeth Licht Publications; 1965.
4. Geddes LA, Silva LF, Dewitt DP, Pearce JA. What's new in electrosurgical instrumentation? Med Instrum. 1977;11:355–61.
5. Stillings D. John Wesley: philosopher of electricity. Med Instrum. 1973;7:307.
6. d'Arsonal A. Action physiologique des courants alternatis a grande frequence. Arch Physiol Porm Pathol. 1893;25:401.
7. Kelly HA, Ward GE. Electrosurgery. Philadelphia: W.B. Saunders; 1932.
8. Doyen E. Sur la destruction des tumeurs cancereuses accessibles: par la methode de la voltaisation bipolaire et de l'electro-coagulation thermique. Arch D'Elecetricitie et de Physiotherapie du Cancer. 1909;17:791–5.
9. Wyeth GA. The endoderm. Am J Electrother Radiol. 1924;42:187.
10. Fervers C. Die laparoskopie mit dem cystoskope. Ein beitrag zur vereinfachung der techniq und aur endoskopischen strangdurchtrennung in der bauchole. Med Klin. 1933;29:1042–5.
11. Power FH, Barnes AC. Sterilization by means of peritoneoscopic fulguration: a preliminary report. Am J Obstet Gynecol. 1941;41:1038–43.
12. Levy BS, Soderstrom RM, Dail DH. Bowel injuries during laparoscopy. Gross anatomy and histology. J Reprod Med. 1985;30:168–72.
13. Frangenheim H. Laparoscopy and culdoscopy in gynaecology. London: Butterworth; 1972.
14. Rioux JE. Bipolar electrosurgery: a short history. J Minim Invasive Gynecol. 2007; 14:538–41.

15. Ohm G. Die galvanische Kette, mathematisch bearbeitet. Berlin: Riemann; 1827.

16. Goldberg SN, Gazelle GS, Halpern EF, Rittman WJ, Mueller PR, Rosenthal DI. Radiofrequency tissue ablation: importance of local temperature along the electrode tip exposure in determining lesion shape and size. Acad Radiol. 1996;3:212–8.

17. Thomsen S. Pathologic analysis of photothermal and photomechanical effects of laser-tissue interactions. Photochem Photobiol. 1991;53:825–35.

18. Lacourse JR, Miller 3rd WT, Vogt M, Selikowitz SM. Effect of high-frequency current on nerve and muscle tissue. IEEE Trans Biomed Eng. 1985;32:82–6.

19. Oringer MJ. Electrosurgery in dentistry. Philadelphia: W.B. Saunders; 1975.

20. Munro MG, Fu YS. Loop electrosurgical excision with a laparoscopic electrode and carbon dioxide laser vaporization: comparison of thermal injury characteristics in the rat uterine horn. Am J Obstet Gynecol. 1995;172:1257–62.

21. Filmar S, Jetha N, McComb P, Gomel VA. A comparative histologic study on the healing process after tissue transection. I. Carbon dioxide laser and electromicrosurgery. Am J Obstet Gynecol. 1989;160:1062–7.

22. Soderstrom RM, Levy BS, Engel T. Reducing bipolar sterilization failures. Obstet Gynecol. 1989;74:60–3.

3. Fundamentals of Electrosurgery Part II: Thermal Injury Mechanisms and Prevention

L. Michael Brunt

It has been estimated that approximately 40,000 patients suffer electrosurgical-related injuries each year [1]. In a survey of members of the American College of Surgeons, 18% of surgeons had experienced insulation failure or a capacitive coupling injury, and 54% knew a colleague who had a stray electrical burn [2]. In laparoscopic surgery, up to 70% of electrosurgical burns may be undetected at the time of injury. As a result, these types of injuries are a frequent source of litigation; indeed, in 1999 nearly $600 million was paid in claims regarding electrosurgical injuries [1].

The death of Congressman John Murtha of Pennsylvania from an intestinal injury during laparoscopic cholecystectomy in 2010 is a cogent reminder of these risks and, therefore, surgeons must be ever vigilant and redouble their efforts to lower the risks associated with electrosurgical energy. In this chapter, the mechanisms of thermal injury are reviewed. Strategies to reduce these risks will also be presented and discussed. In addition, the hazards of electrosurgical-related smoke and smoke injuries and electrosurgery-induced fires are presented.

Mechanisms of Electrosurgical Injury

The various mechanisms by which electrosurgical injuries may occur are listed in Table 3.1. These include injuries at the dispersive electrode site (previously known as the patient ground pad or "Bovie" pad), injuries due to current diversion to an unintended site, and active electrode injuries that may result from either inadvertent activation or direct extension.

L.S. Feldman et al. (eds.), *The SAGES Manual on the Fundamental Use of Surgical Energy (FUSE)*, DOI 10.1007/978-1-4614-2074-3_3, © Springer Science+Business Media, LLC 2012

Table 3.1. Mechanisms of electrosurgical injury.

Dispersive electrode
  Application site issues
  Partial detachment

Current diversion
  Insulation failure
  Direct coupling
  Capacitive coupling
  Alternate site injuries

Active electrode Injury
  Inadvertent activation
  Direct extension

Some basic patient protection measures should be undertaken for the electrosurgical unit (ESU) itself. The ESU should be inspected periodically for any external damage. No fluids should be placed on top of the ESU, and it should never be used in the presence of flammable materials (e.g., alcohol, nitrous oxide). The lowest possible power settings should be used that will deliver the desired thermal effect to the patient tissues. In the presence of tissue edema (whether from acute inflammation or locally infiltrated anesthetic), higher power settings may be necessary to achieve the desired effect, since the water in the tissue must first be vaporized before the target tissue is affected. Activation and indicator alarms should be loud enough so that they can be easily heard over the background or ambient noise in the room. In many operating rooms, music is often played during the surgical case, and the volume of the music must be balanced with the ability to readily hear these alarms. Surgeons and nursing personnel should also work together to establish a mechanism for confirming and communicating power settings before starting the case and verifying any changes that occur during the case. For example, if the surgeon says "increase the coagulation power to 50 W," the nurse should reply "coagulation power at 50" and the surgeon should respond with a "thank you" or other affirmation that he/she has understood that the requested changes were made.

Dispersive Electrode

It is important to ensure that the patient is not in direct contact with any metal objects and is on an insulated table. Older grounded-type generators would allow return of current through any conductor that is in contact with earth. For example, if the patient's arm were in contact with a metal post, then the current would pass through the patient into that post, potentially resulting in a burn to the patient at the contact point with the post. The current generation of systems with isolated circuits has essentially eliminated this possibility because all elements in the circuit are in continuity with the generator itself and are grounded through the generator. In other words, if the current leaves the patient by a site other than the dispersive electrode, the reduced current in the circuit is recognized by the generator, prompting it to automatically shut off delivery of any further current to the system, including the active electrode [3]. It is also advisable for all jewelry to be removed from the patient for a variety of reasons, although with isolated generator technology it is not necessary due to electrosurgical considerations only. Any jewelry that is potentially in the direct path of ES current (e.g., tongue ring for tonsillectomy procedure), however, should be removed. Likewise, direct contact of the active electrode or ES cord with jewelry should be avoided [4].

A schematic illustration of dispersive electrode physics is shown in Fig. 3.1. For a monopolar electrosurgical instrument, the active electrode site has a small contact area with high current (or power) density which creates the thermal effect. In contrast, the dispersive electrode has a large surface area that results in a low current density at any given site [3]. In order for the dispersive electrode to function properly, the contact with the patient must be uniform over a large surface area. Therefore, the following areas should be avoided: bony prominences, metal implants or prosthesis, scar tissue, hairy areas, areas adjacent to leads/electrodes, pressure areas/points, and skin discoloration/injury or limbs with circulatory compromise. The dispersive electrode should *never* be cut to size. Once the dispersive electrode has been removed for any reason, it must be replaced by a new pad. The dispersive electrode should be placed as close as possible to the active surgical site in order to minimize current effects to other areas of the body. Finally, no hardware should be interspersed between the active electrode and the dispersive electrode (e.g., hip prosthesis, cardiac implanted electrical device).

Most modern ESUs are capable of utilizing a split dispersive electrode (Fig. 3.2). The split dispersive electrode design allows the ESU to monitor impedance both in total and in each of the split portions of the dispersive electrode. If the split dispersive electrode detaches even partially, a difference in the measured impedance between the split electrodes will prompt the ESU to shut off. This gives additional protection to the patient in case the dispersive electrode is placed over an

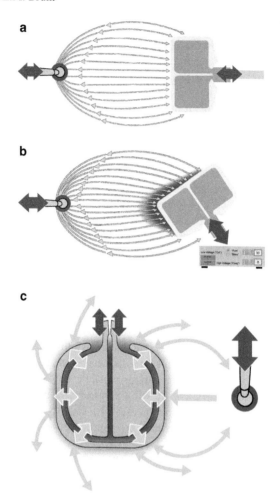

Fig. 3.1. (**a–c**) Schematic illustration of dispersive electrode physics. A monopolar system includes two electrodes, with the patient in between. The active electrode shown on the right is small in order to focus the current from the ESU and create the desired tissue effect while the second, large electrode shown on the left is placed remotely on the patient to disperse the current. Because of the relatively large surface area of the dispersive electrode, the current at any given site is low and does not result in any thermal effect at that site.

area of poor conductivity or becomes partially detached. Obese patients, because there is greater impedance in adipose tissue, may require a second dispersive electrode [5]. The second electrode may be placed on the same or opposite thigh, arm, leg, or flank.

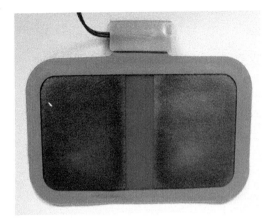

Fig. 3.2. Split return design of the dispersive electrode. The generator shuts off if current is not uniformly returned to the generator across the two pads.

Current Diversion

Insulation Failure

Insulation failure may be a source of electrosurgical injury during laparoscopic procedures. The smaller the break in the insulation, the higher the current density will be at that defective insulation site as the current is focused over a very small area. These breaks are often invisible to the naked eye, even with careful inspection. Therefore, active electrode monitoring systems to screen instruments for insulation breaks have been designed [6] and can be very useful in identifying breaks that are not readily apparent to the user (Fig. 3.3). All insulated electrosurgical instruments should undergo regular active monitoring for insulation breaks.

Direct Coupling

Direct coupling occurs when one conductive element of the circuit touches or arcs to an instrument outside of the intended circuit. Direct coupling is often intentionally utilized intraoperatively for coagulation purposes. For example, a monopolar electrosurgical instrument is held in contact with a forceps in order to coagulate small bleeders as shown in Fig. 3.4. In laparoscopic surgery, this approach carries the risk of inadvertently directing the current toward nontargeted tissue (bowel or

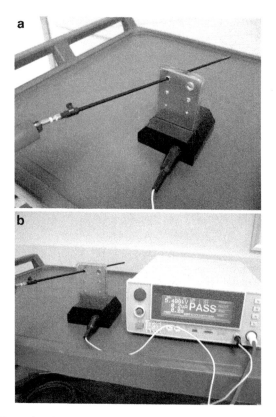

Fig. 3.3. Example of one type of active electrode monitoring system used to detect insulation failure in laparoscopic instruments. (**a**) The instrument is passed back and forth through a test plate while connected to the monitoring unit. (**b**) The "PASS" readout on the monitoring unit indicates that no insulation breaks were detected. If a break was present, the readout would have been "FAIL".

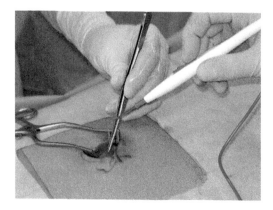

Fig. 3.4. Example of direct coupling from a monopolar device to a forceps.

the abdominal wall) [7], especially if the view of the instrument in contact with the active electrode is partially or completely obscured. Finally, the surgeon may be at risk for personal injury. If the monopolar instrument is activated at the proximal end of the forceps above the surgeon's hand and not near the tip of the forceps in contact with the tissue, the current must pass along the part of the instrument where the surgeon's hand is in contact with it; if there is a break in the glove or prolonged activation leading to high current density and breakdown of the glove, the surgeon's hand may be burned.

Capacitive Coupling

Capacitance is defined as stored electrical charge when two conductors are separated by a nonconductive dielectric, also called an insulator [3]. Capacitive coupling occurs when the circuit is completed through the dielectric. Charge will be stored in the capacitor until either the generator is deactivated or a pathway to complete the circuit is achieved (Fig. 3.5). By its very nature, capacitive coupling can occur only with the use of monopolar instrumentation. It is not a risk with bipolar instruments because current passes only between the two tips of the active electrodes.

The amount of capacitance and the subsequent risk of capacitive coupling are related to the length of the cannula (L), radius of the cannula (b), radius of the active electrode (a), and dielectric constant of the insulator (k) [3]. This relationship is expressed by the formula $C = L/2 k \ln(b/a)$. Factors that increase the risk of capacitive coupling include (1) high voltage waveform ("coagulation" output); (2) ratio of the

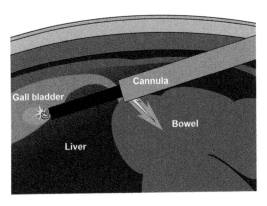

Fig. 3.5. Schematic illustration of capacitive coupling. For details see text.

electrosurgical instrument's outside diameter to that of the laparoscopic cannula or port (risk is greater with 5 mm than 11 mm ports); (3) activation over previously desiccated tissue due to the high resistance to current flow; and (4) "open" activation of the system, i.e., activation of the electrode before it becomes in contact with the tissue, which increases the voltage. This phenomenon may occur in a laparoscopic case if the monopolar electrosurgical instrument used to dissect the gallbladder is activated several centimeters before making contact with the tissue.

Prior to the development of small video cameras suitable for endoscopic use, surgeons performed laparoscopy by looking directly down the eyepiece of the scope. As a result, burns to the eye would occasionally occur due to the capacitive charge that would build up within the laparoscope and metal cannula through which it passed. Capacitive coupling may also occur when the electrosurgical (ES) cable is wrapped around a metal instrument (e.g., metal clamp on the surgical drapes) or is in close proximity to a metal total hip prosthesis. The use of multiple ES devices simultaneously (either two monopolar or one monopolar and one bipolar device) may also lead to capacitive charge buildup. Precautions in this setting include keeping the two cords separate and avoid attaching them in close proximity to one another or looped together around a towel clip or clamp [8].

Others situations where the risk of capacitive coupling increases include the use of a wet, insulated monopolar instrument or, less commonly, when a metal cannula is used with a plastic abdominal anchor. Although such plastic grips or anchors are rarely utilized anymore, they can greatly increase the risk capacitance because the plastic insulates the abdominal wall from current and, therefore, allows the creation of a capacitive charge on the cannula. This charge is then capable of arcing to adjacent abdominal viscera [7, 9].

Alternate Site Injuries

Because current is delivered to the patient through a circuit that includes the electrosurgical generator (ESU), current diversion may occur when elements of the circuit interface with any conductive structure, a circumstance that can cause injury. This phenomenon is much less common with today's ESUs as they will automatically shut down if the unit detects reduced current flow because of an alternate current pathway. Nonetheless, basic precautions should be employed to prevent patient contact with any metal or other objects with high conductivity as discussed previously.

Active Electrode Injury

Inadvertent Activation

A relatively common cause of active electrode-related injury is inadvertent activation. This may occur with any handheld monopolar instrument including those used for laparoscopic surgery. For this reason, the handheld ES monopolar "pencil" should never be placed on the patient's skin or on the drapes over the face or chest when not in use (Fig. 3.6), but instead should always be replaced in the plastic holster. Inadvertent activation of an ES device is especially dangerous during laparoscopic cases when the activation control is through a foot pedal on the operating room floor and structures near the active electrode tip (e.g., intestine) may be out of the field of view. An example of this phenomenon is illustrated in Fig. 3.7. In this scenario, a monopolar instrument is placed into the laparoscopic surgical field and the surgeon looks away from the field to locate the foot pedal to activate the device. Meanwhile, the tip of the instrument is not sheathed in the port but is inside the abdominal cavity and the tip is out of the field of view; it may even be very close to or in direct contact with the intestine or other viscera. As the surgeon looks away, the instruments position may shift further. If inadvertent activation of the foot pedal were to occur, this could result in a thermal injury that is out of view and undetected and could potentially cause a delayed intestinal perforation with serious consequences. Special care should also be taken when dual ES systems are simultaneously in use (e.g., two monopolar instruments) to avoid unintentional activation of the wrong device.

Direct Thermal Extension

Direct thermal extension may occur when one structure is near or attached to the other by an adhesion or other segment of tissue. Adhesions between the gallbladder and duodenum, especially if the attachment to the duodenum is narrow, can put the duodenum at increased risk for thermal injury if electrosurgery is used to divide the adhesion. This risk is further increased with prolonged activation or reapplication of energy to tissue that has already been desiccated with an initial ES application [3]. Many biliary injuries during laparoscopic cholecystectomy also involve a component of electrosurgical injury. While most of these are misidentification injuries and are not exclusively related to use of electrosurgery, the common bile duct and right hepatic artery are

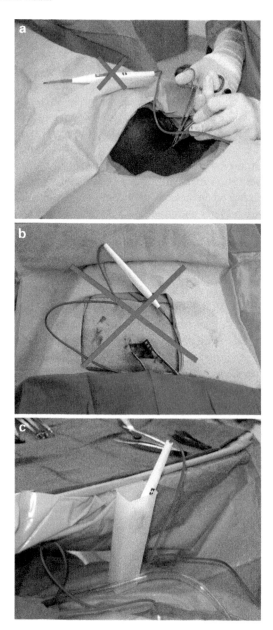

Fig. 3.6. (**a, b**) Improper placement of monopolar ES pencil on top of surgical drapes in area of patient's face or in direct contact with the skin. (**c**) Active ES tips should always be returned to a protective holder when not in use.

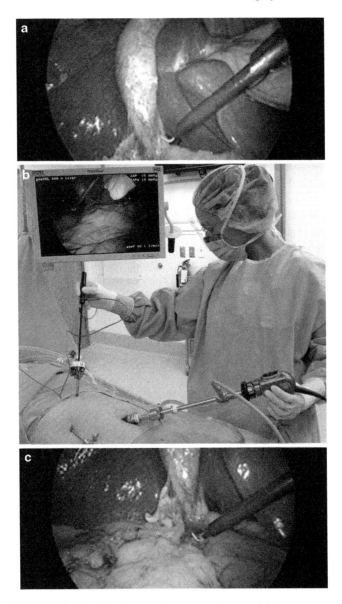

Fig. 3.7. (**a–c**) Risks of inadvertent electrode activation. (**a**) Active monopolar hook instrument is positioned within the peritoneal cavity to dissect the gallbladder. (**b**) Surgeon looks away from the field to locate activation foot pedal. (**c**) Monopolar tip drifts away into a position near or in contact with the duodenum. Inadvertent activation at this point could create an intestinal injury out of the field of view that could result in delayed perforation.

nonetheless vulnerable to thermal injury because of their proximity to the hepatocystic triangle. Short activations of the electrode of no more than 2–3 s at a time are recommended to minimize the risk for above types of injuries.

Surgeons are also at risk for electrosurgical injuries from direct extension. Holes are present in approximately 15% of new surgical gloves and in up to 50% after use in the operating room [3]. Capacitive coupling injuries may also occur from sweating inside the surgical glove. High voltages across the glove may break the insulating capacity of the glove and lead to an injury. Glove resistance is also decreased with time and exposure to saline (e.g., sweating). The risk of a capacitive coupling injury through a surgical glove is inversely proportional to the glove's thickness and increases with higher voltage and longer contact time. For example, the longer the electrode is activated while touching a hemostatic clamp held by the surgeon, the greater the risk of injury. Activating the electrode in the air and then touching a hemostat may also increase the risk of a thermal injury to the surgeon. Similarly, in laparoscopic surgery, it is advisable to use fully insulated instruments so that the surgeon's hand is not in contact with any exposed metal while holding the instrument (Fig. 3.8).

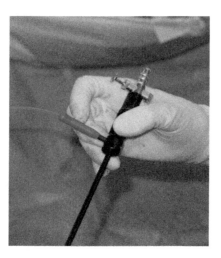

Fig. 3.8. Surgeon's hand in direct contact with metal conductor on a monopolar laparoscopic hook device, which may enhance the risk of a burn to the surgeon's hand.

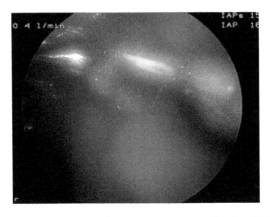

Fig. 3.9. Electrosurgical smoke is a common cause of reduced visualization during laparoscopic surgery.

Electrosurgery and Smoke

Smoke is a byproduct of any electrosurgical device. The most obvious adverse effect of smoke in the operating room is interference with laparoscopic visualization (Fig. 3.9). Both passive and active laparoscopic evacuation and filtration systems have been designed to minimize the interference of smoke plume with visualization of the operative field. However, none of the currently available systems have provided a completely satisfactory solution to this problem, and surgeons must be careful to maintain the visualization necessary for safe dissection and operation of energy devices. In general, short activation sequences result in less extensive smoke plumes and less clouding of the visual field.

An additional consideration is the by-products of electrosurgical vaporization that are contained in the smoke plume [10] that may include toxic vapors and gases such as benzene, hydrogen cyanide and form-aldehyde, chemicals and irritants including some that are potentially mutagenic or carcinogenic, bioaerosols including blood fragments, viruses and viral particles, and, in laparoscopic surgery, methemoglobin and carboxyhemoglobin [11]. Surgical masks only filter particles down to approximately 5 μm whereas 77% of surgical smoke contents are 1.1 μm or smaller [12].

High concentrations of smoke have been shown to occasionally cause ocular and upper respiratory irritation in healthcare personnel [13].

However, there has been no documentation of cancer cases from smoke exposure in the OR. A number of strategies have been utilized to reduce smoke exposure in the operating room. These include central smoke evacuation systems, portable smoke evacuation units, wall suction with in line filters, and, as mentioned above, laparoscopic evacuation filtration systems. Suction clearance of the smoke plume has been shown to reduce the amount of smoke reaching the level of the surgeon's mask [14], but the smoke should be evacuated within 1 inch of the source, otherwise only 50% or less will be evacuated [15]. An efficient smoke evacuation system should have a capture device which does not impede the surgeon's conduct of the procedure, a vacuum source strong enough to remove the smoke properly, and a filtration system that has adequate filtration capability. The Occupational Safety and Health Administration (OSHA) and Association of peri-Operative Registered Nurses (AORN) have both recommended that smoke evacuation systems should be used to reduce acute and chronic risks to patients and to healthcare personnel [16, 17]. AORN has also developed practice recommendations to assist in the selection of smoke evacuation systems [18].

Fires and Explosions

Fires and explosions are rare but potentially devastating events in the operating room. Explosion risk has been reduced significantly from the era of ether and cyclopropane anesthesia prior to the 1970s when these anesthetic gases were commonly utilized. Another potential source of explosive gas is from the gastrointestinal tract. The bowel contains hydrogen-air mixtures between 4 and 7% and methane between 5 and 15% [3]. Mannitol promotes the production of methane and, therefore, is contraindicated for bowel preparation prior to surgery [19]. The use of nitrous oxide also enhances the risk for the formation of a potentially explosive combination of gases.

Fires in the operating room are rare, but the ECRI has estimated that between 550 and 650 operating room fires occur each year. These numbers equal those of wrong-site surgery cases per year. Approximately 95% of these fires are minor and result in no injury. However, each year 20–30 OR fire-related injuries are associated with disfiguring or disabling outcomes. In 2003, the Joint Commission issued a sentinel event alert on preventing surgical fires [20]. Surgical fire prevention is also 1 of the 11 priority safety topics identified by the Association of peri-Operative Registered Nurses (AORN) Presidential Commission on Patient Safety [21]. AORN has also developed a fire safety tool kit [22], and the Anesthesia Patient Safety Foundation has developed an educational video on fire risk in the OR [23].

In order for a fire to occur, three elements must be present as illustrated in the fire triangle in Fig. 3.10. These three elements are (1) a heat or ignition source which is usually from the ESU or surgical lasers; (2) fuel which consists of the surgical drapes and/or surgical prep material; and (3) an oxidizer (O_2, N_2O). Prevention of OR fires requires an awareness of the risk factors and coordination by the healthcare providers.

According to data from the ECRI Institute, approximately 21% of surgical fires occur in the airway, 44% around the head, neck, face, or upper chest, and the remainder elsewhere [20]. About 70% are on the patient and just under 30% in the patient, most commonly within the airway. In the majority of cases (70%), the ignition source is the electrosurgical equipment. The remainder are caused by surgical lasers (c. 10% of cases) and other equipment such as fiber optic light sources. Lasers may be an especially potent source for fire ignition since they can

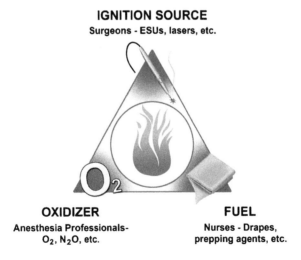

IGNITION SOURCE
Surgeons - ESUs, lasers, etc.

OXIDIZER
Anesthesia Professionals-
O_2, N_2O, etc.

FUEL
Nurses - Drapes,
prepping agents, etc.

Fig. 3.10. Fire triangle. The three elements that are necessary for a surgical fire to develop are an oxidizer (e.g., oxygen), fuel (surgical drapes, surgical prep solutions), and an igniter or heat source (ES energy or laser). (We thank ECRI Institute for the concepts used for design of the surgical fire triangle graphic. Free resources on surgical fire prevention are available at www.ecri.org/surgical_fires).

burn through drapes and other objects in their path [24]. The ECRI institute has published guidelines "Only You can Prevent Surgical Fires" which highlights the importance of surgical team communication [20]. Some of the key preventive strategies include minimizing the use of open oxygen sources (i.e., via a mask or cannula) for head and neck procedures. When performing a tracheostomy, the surgeon should use cold instruments on the tracheal rings to enter the surgical airway because of the oxygen present in the airway. One must be aware of O_2 enrichment under the surgical drapes, especially during head and neck procedures. Surgical drapes should not be applied until flammable preps or alcohol-based preps have fully dried, and any spilled or pooled material should be soaked up prior to starting the procedure. Note that alcohol based fires may not be immediately apparent due to the colorless or dim blue flame produced by burning alcohol. Water-based betadine scrub is not flammable, although tinctures of betadine or iodine which contain alcohol are. Fiber optic light cables should be connected before the source is activated and should subsequently be placed on standby before disconnecting or placing the scope onto the surgical drapes.

The entire team should be aware whenever open O_2 is in use, by including it into the preoperative checklist and team discussion. The ESU should only be activated when the tip of the active electrode is in view and should be deactivated before the active electrode leaves the surgical site. As noted above, it is extremely important that the ES device be placed in a plastic holster when not in use. It should never be placed upon the patient's chest, face, or groin region. In addition, rubber sleeves should not be used over ES electrodes because they are not insulators and can cause flame flare-ups, especially in O_2-rich environments.

In the event that a fire does occur in the operating room, a number of steps should be immediately undertaken. First, the flow of all airway gases to the patient should be stopped and the patient should be disconnected from the breathing circuit. If the fire is in the airway, the breathing circuit should be disconnected from the tube and the endotracheal tube should be immediately removed. Second, any burning and burned materials, whether on or in the patient, should be immediately removed. Third, the fire should be extinguished from the burning materials. Usually this can be done by smothering the fire or dousing it with saline. The use of a CO_2 fire extinguisher is rarely necessary unless the fire has engulfed the patient, involves materials that continue to burn after removal from the patient, or has spread off the patient or involves OR equipment [20]. Step 4 consists of resumption of care for the patient. Breathing should be restored using room air and never with oxygen, and patient burn injuries should be managed in a standard manner. In the event of disastrous or extreme smoke and fire conditions, the steps should follow the **RACE** acronym: **Rescue**, Alert, Confine, and Evacuate [20]. In the **Rescue** phase, attempts should be made to rescue the patient from the fire in the operating room. Staff should be **Alerted** and fire alarm systems should be activated and the fire department called as indicated. The room should be **Confined** including closing all doors, and shutting off medical gas valves, automatic smoke evacuations, and electrical power to the room. The incident room in which the fire has occurred should be **Evacuated** and, if necessary, the entire operating room suite should be evacuated. Over the last 30 plus years, there have been only two known cases in which the operating room had to be evacuated due to a surgical fire, and in only one of these cases was a burning patient left behind. For further information on this topic, the reader is referred to one of a number of guidelines for OR fire prevention that have been published by various professional societies [23, 25, 26] as well as the nonprofit patient safety research group, the ECRI Institute [20].

OR Fire

Operating room fire is an uncommon but devastating problem. More than 600 fires occur in operating rooms in the United States yearly. Many of these fires result in serious injury and even death. About a quarter of operating room fires do NOT involve the face, head or neck. It is unlikely that any of those burned patients were apprised of, or seriously concerned about, fire as a potential complication of their procedure as they were wheeled into the operating room and placed on the table. The lay press has drawn attention to these tragedies on the Internet, complete with before and after photographs that illustrate the magnitude of the devastation inflicted upon patients who often felt they were to undergo a "simple" procedure [27].

Surgeons, nurses, technicians and anesthesia personnel must be educated, then committed and vigilant in order to achieve the ZERO FIRE goal. The components of the *fire triangle* of fuel, oxidizer, and ignition must not be allowed to come together. In order to achieve this, OR team communication is essential - first by assessing fire risk for each case during the safety checklist and throughout the case where hazards may exist. Meticulous surgical technique that eliminates sparking in hazardous conditions and unintended electrosurgical unit activation is also an absolute requirement if this goal is to be reached. The public expects and deserves nothing less. (S.D. Schwaitzberg, MD, FACS, SAGES President 2010–2011).

Summary

In summary, surgeons who work with electrosurgical equipment should be knowledgeable about the basic principles of electrosurgery, risks to patients and personnel, and measures to minimize these risks. They should be aware of the hazards associated with smoke in the OR environment and should understand the factors that can lead to OR fires and the proper corrective actions to be taken in the event of a fire or electrosurgical-related injury.

References

1. Lee J. Update on electrosurgery. Outpatient Surg. 2002;2(2):44–53.
2. Tucker RD. Laparoscopic electrosurgical injuries: survey results and their implications. Surg Laparosc Endosc. 1995;5:311–7.
3. Amaral JF. Electrosurgery and ultrasound for cutting and coagulating tissue in minimally invasive surgery. In: Soper NJ, Swanstrom LL, Eubanks WS, editors. Mastery of endoscopic and laparoscopic surgery. Philadelphia: Lippincott, Wilkins, Williams; 2005. p. 67–82.
4. Fickling J, Leoeffler CR. Body jewelry—to remove of not remove, that is the question. Clin Inform Hotline. 2000; clincial.hotline@valleylab.com.
5. Conner R. Dual return electrodes; electrosurgical fires, fluid biohazards; cleaning alcohol; free-flowing oxygen. AORN J. 2003;77:1012–8.
6. Vancaille TG. Active electrode monitoring: how to prevent unintentional thermal injury associated with electrosurgery at laparoscopy. Surg Endosc. 1998;12:1009–12.
7. Newman RM, Traverso LW. Principles of laparoscopic hemostasis. In: Scott-Connor CEH, editor. The SAGES manual: fundamentals of laparoscopy, thoracoscopy, and GI endoscopy. New York: Springer; 2006. p. 49–59.
8. Vilos G, Latendresse K, Gan BS. Electrophysical properties of electrosurgery and capacitive induced current. Am J Surg. 2001;182:222–5.
9. Tucker RD, Platz CE, Landas SK. A laparoscopic complication? A medical legal case analysis. J Gynecol Surg. 1995;11:185–92.
10. Hollmann R, Hort CE, Kammer E, Naegele M, Sigrist MW, Meuli-Simmen C. Smoke in the operating theater: an unregarded danger. Plast Reconstr Surg. 2004;114: 458–63.

11. Recommended practices for electrosurgery. AORN J. 2005;81:616–42.
12. Stanton C. Taking a stand on surgical smoke. AORN Connections 2008. http://www.aorn. org/News/April2008News/TakingaStandOnSurgicalSmoke/. Accessed 31 Aug 2011.
13. OSHA. Control of smoke from laser/electric surgical procedures. DHHS (NIOSH) publication 96–128. Atlanta: National Institute for Occupational Safety and Health; 1996.
14. Pillinger SH, Delbridge L, Lewis DR. Randomized clinical trial of suction verse standard clearance of the diathermy plume. Br J Surg. 2003;90:1068–71.
15. Biggins J, Renfree S. The hazards of surgical smoke are not to be sniffed at. Br J Perioper Nurs. 2002;12(4):136–8; 141–3.
16. Statement O. Lasers and electrosurgery plume. http://wwwoshagov/SLTC/laserelectro- surgeryplume/indexhtml. Accessed 2011.
17. AORN Position Statement. http://wwwaornorg/PracticeResources/AORNPosition Statements/SurgicalSmokeAndBioAerosols/. Accessed 2011.
18. Aorn I. Recommended practices for product selection in perioperative practice settings. In: Aorn I, editor. Standards, recommended practices, and guidelines. Denver: Assn of Operating Room Nurses; 2004. p. 347–50.
19. Avgerinos A, Kalantzis N, Rekoumis G, et al. Bowel preparation and the risk of explosion during colonic polypectomy. Gut. 1984;25:361–4.
20. ECRI Institute. New clinical guide to surgical fire prevention. Health Devices. 2009; 38(10):314–22.
21. Beyea SC. Preventing fires in the OR. AORN J. 2003;78:664–6.
22. AORN. Fire safety tool kit. http://wwwaornorg/PracticeResources/ToolKits/FireSafety ToolKit/2010. Accessed 31 Aug 2011.
23. Anesthesia Patient Safety Foundation. Prevention and management of surgical fires (video). http://wwwapsforg/resource_center/educationaltools/video_librarymspx. Accessed 31 Aug 2011.
24. Podnos YD, Williams RA. Fires in the operating room. Bull Am Coll Surg. 1997; 82:14–7.
25. American Society of Anesthesiology. Task force on operating room fires. Anesthesiology. 2008;108:768–801.
26. Statement AG. Fire prevention in the operating room. AORN. 2005;81:1067–75.
27. Aleccia, J. On fire in the OR: Hundreds are hurt every year. http://today.msnbc.msn.com/ id/26874567/ns/today-today_health/t/fire-or-hundreds-are-hurt-every-year/?ns=health- health_care&t=fire-or-hundreds-are-hurt-every-year. Accessed 1 Dec 2010.

4. The Art and Science of Monopolar Electrosurgery

C. Randle Voyles

Background

The concepts introduced herein are not new. Indeed, the biophysical principles were well described almost 90 years ago. While many investigators made early contributions, perhaps the best materials were written by Cushing and Bovie [1]. Additionally, a wonderful text was written in 1932 from the Hopkins early experience and investigations [2]. The acronomial relationship of $\Delta t \, \alpha \, (I^2/A^2)R\,T$ is unique to this publication but is a direct extrapolation of the above works. The potential problems with laparoscopic electrosurgery were described by many investigators; the author's early work including zones of injury in general surgery is referenced [3]. The following comments about single port laparoscopy are not yet published but represent simple extrapolation of earlier work. The potential problems with argon beam are well outlined [4, 5].

First Things First

The most polished application of an energy source is an art form with the stroke of the monopolar electrode, not unlike that of the most renowned artist. Yes, our canvas is perhaps more dynamic as are our outcomes. For the artist confined to the constraints of a canvas, the beauty of the end result is in the eye of the beholder. For the surgical artist, the only real-time beholder may only be the surgeon but subsequent quality measures (observed by by-standing "beholders") might include less pain, less bleeding, early discharge, shorter operating times, uneventful recovery, and likely lower costs, or alternatively, the need for transfusion, morbidity, and perhaps even mortality.

L.S. Feldman et al. (eds.), *The SAGES Manual on the Fundamental Use of Surgical Energy (FUSE)*, DOI 10.1007/978-1-4614-2074-3_4, © Springer Science+Business Media, LLC 2012

The traditional artist employs a variety of mechanical strokes and paints to initiate visual change on the canvas. In a similar fashion, the electrosurgical artist also employs varying techniques and tools to initiate visual change on a tissue canvas. The traditional artists and the electrosurgical artist anticipate the effect of minor modifications of technique. It is a tribute to the ease of use of basic monopolar electrosurgery that its application has been so successful with a very limited understanding of the underlying biophysics by the end-using surgeon. Indeed, surgical application has been accomplished traditionally by intuitive learning ("see one, do one, teach one"). However, a basic understanding is a prerequisite to an improved art form. Furthermore, technical challenges with increasingly complex biophysical contortions of instrumentation mandate a better understanding of elementary biophysics (as outlined in the two previous chapters).

Second Things Second

All of the tissue effects of monopolar electrosurgery are primarily a direct result of thermal change. Thus it behooves the surgeon to understand some of the principles of thermal change. What are the variables that initiate thermal change? How is it controlled? Three goals of application are definable:

1. Limited thermal change to target tissue *only*
2. Adequate hemostasis
3. Tissue cutting/vaporization/transection

In an effort to maximize these goals, intuition alone is insufficient. The science of the effort is fairly easy to understand, albeit a bit more difficult to master. The following discourse is outlined not from the view of the extraneously detailed biophysicist but rather from the practicing surgeon who asks "what do I need to know?"

Third Things Third

$$\text{Current density} = \frac{\text{Current } (I)}{\text{Area } (A)}$$

As outlined in previous chapters, the patient is part of the completed electrical circuit as the current alternates between the active electrode and the dispersive electrode (previously referred to as the return pad). The goal of the electrosurgeon is to concentrate the current (represented by the letter "I") only at the target tissue and avoid concentration at all other points of the circuit. Thus, there is just as much current at the active electrode as at the dispersive electrode; the latter pad provides a large area for dispersion and accordingly, very little thermal change (Δt). Thermal change (Δt) $\propto$ current density^2.

$$\Delta T \propto I^2 / A^2$$

Thermal change *at every point in the circuit* is a function of current density *squared*. As Goal #1 is to avoid thermal change to nontarget tissue, it behooves the surgeon to keep the current as low as possible and exploit the biophysics of focusing the current to as small an area as possible. Take-home point: Do not turn up the wattage (which will increase the "I"); instead, maximize the benefit of concentrating current (by decreasing the "A"). Here is an example to make the point.

In Fig. 4.1, an articulating electrode is shown touching the target tissue: in the left image with two tines, in the right image with only one. What is the difference in "tissue thermal change" in each scenario? Assuming the same "I" in each, the second model has half the area or "A." Furthermore, since $A = \pi r^2$, it follows:

$$\Delta T \propto I^2 / r^4$$

$$\tfrac{1}{2}\ \text{radius} \propto 16\,\Delta T$$

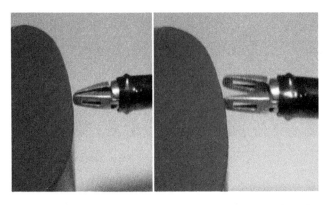

Fig. 4.1. An articulating electrode is shown touching the target tissue in the *left image* with two tines, and in the *right image* with only one.

For practical purposes, there is a 16-fold increase in thermal change with reduction of radius by half. (Practicing surgeons recognize the impact of this relationship when using needle electrodes but may not be familiar with the mathematical relationship.) The academic biophysicist may argue some points but the take-home message is to use fine electrodes with limited contact with tissue in order to exploit this message of applied biophsics. Refrain from simply increasing the wattage output from the generator (in order to increase "I") as previously outined.

The final two variables include resistance ("R") at each point within the circuit and time ("T"), respectively, that complete the formula for ΔT. Thermal change increases in a linear fashion with tissue resistance ($\Delta T \propto R^1$). Tissue resistance may be increased by removing conductive fluid (blood), compressing arteries or putting tissue under stretch. Also, doubling the *time* of application doubles the thermal change in a corresponding linear relationship ($\Delta T \propto t^1$). Putting the science of the art in a formula discloses a useful acronomial relationship (Fig. 4.2).

The practical minded surgical artist implements the science of the ART through the *ART* of the science exploiting what he/she knows to be most efficacious (change first the big "A" as it is the highest powered useful function and then the "R" and "t") and avoiding the fallback position of increasing the "I" with the associated increased risks of unwanted thermal change. (*As an aside, why is current measured in amperes represented by "I?" It is suggested that "I" may have come from "intensity" but for teaching purposes, perhaps it should represent "ill-advised" or "inappropriate." Go for the ART and not the inappropriate*).

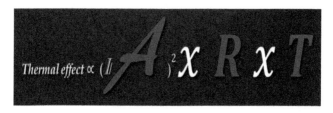

Fig. 4.2. Putting the science of the art in a formula discloses a useful acronomial relationship.

Which Electrodes Should I Use?

Hooks and spatulas are the simplest and easiest electrodes for learning purposes. The ART formula suggests that the electrode should have a quite fine edge for some purposes as well as a broad surface for fulguration and coaptation. After mastering elementary concepts, the skilled electrosurgeon finds that the articulating electrodes shown in Fig. 4.3a offer all of the benefits of a hook with many additional functions: reaching around a curve (Fig. 4.3b), enhanced dissection of fine tissues (Fig. 4.3e), and grasping coaptation of structures (Fig. 4.3f). The primary disadvantage of the articulating device (exposure of metal of the working end) can be overcome by a simple adjustable sleeve (Fig. 4.3c, d).

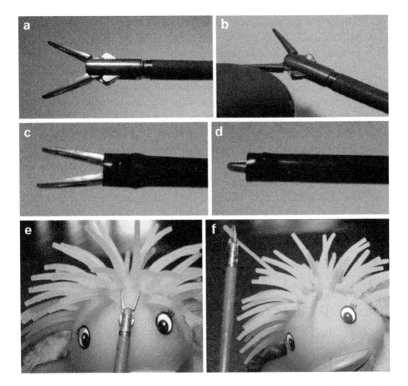

Fig. 4.3. The articulating electrodes shown in (**a**) offer all of the benefits of a hook with many additional functions: reaching around a curve (**b**), enhanced dissection of fine tissues (**e**), and grasping coaptation of structures (**f**). The primary disadvantage of the articulating device (exposure of metal of the working end) can be overcome by a simple adjustable sleeve (**c**, **d**).

How Do I Assess the Efficacy and Safety of My Electrosurgical Surgical Technique?

The three aforementioned goals of limited thermal change, effective hemostasis, and tissue transection are not arguable. However, surgical technique varies from surgeon to surgeon. However, most should agree that the ESU wattage should be as low as possible to accomplish the task. The use of a very low wattage (i.e., 20 W power) forces the surgeon to exploit the "ART" portion of the formula. "*A*" is exploited by using the fine edge of the electrode with limited tissue contact but more so through superb traction and tension on tissue. (Reread the paragraph and concentrate for a moment on the combination of understanding the science and applying the art).

There is visible "qualitative" evidence of thermal change in the target (and nontarget) tissue. Water boils at 100°C. Tissue turns to a tan color with desiccation and protein denaturation at a range of 70–150°C. Tissue turns black with carbonization at temperatures from 200 to 400°C. Carbonization is frequently a manifestation of poor exposure, poor countertension, and poor hemostasis; thus, blackened tissue is generally not a hallmark of meticulous dissection. Black carbonized tissue may be tolerated in selected "safe" areas away from vital structures. However, the gallbladder bed is not "safe" as the bed often contains very superficially located segmental ducts and vessels. (Most laparoscopic residents in general surgery learn to use electrosurgery with cholecystectomy. Upon completion of the resection, the surgeon should assess collateral thermal damage to the gallbladder bed: black should be avoided and tan discoloration should be minimized).

A Practical Questions About Metal-to-Metal Arcing: What Is the Highest Temperature that Can Be Created During a Laparoscopic Procedure?

The answer is over 1,000°C. How so? In "normal circumstance" when an active electrode touches biologic tissue, desiccation impairs current flow and thus limits current concentration and temperature change. Accordingly, to create an excessively high temperature (previous paragraphs), one must have a continuous high current ("*I*") with the lowest area ("*A*") of contact. How is current maintained with such a low area? The answer: A metal staple line. Given adequate wattage to maintain a continuous arc to an isolated staple (as may occur when the surgeon fulgurates a bleeding staple line), the row of metal staples creates a low resistance pathway that allows the current to increase dramatically. Given a continuous arc between active electrode and staple, the area of the arc is the smallest possible "*A*." Enough heat can be generated in the pathway to melt the exposed staple, which occurs at 1,000° and transfers the heat to adjacent biologic tissue (See Fig. 15.1). Message: Use utmost care with energy sources around metal clips and staples. "Buzzing" a staple line may lead to delayed and unrecognized tissue breakdown and anastomotic leak.

Metal to metal arcing can also occur between the active electrode and other metal instruments (clips, graspers, laparoscope, and cannulas). While larger metal instruments generally will not "melt" like a staple line, the intermittent arcing process of the current from metal to metal can create bursts of lower frequency currents that provide a unique interference with the video monitor (creating "lightning artifacts") as well as neuromuscular stimulation with focal jerking of the abdominal wall (particulary when using metal cannulas) due to lower frequency currents; these lower frequency currents (often referred to as "demodulated currents") may cause tetanic contraction of voluntary muscle (often referred to as the "faradic effect"). The surgeon should be cognizant of the subtle findings of metal to metal arcing, for these same subtle effects may represent clues to stray currents of insulation failure and direct coupling.

What Are the Factors Unique to Monopolar Electrosurgery?

Perhaps the most distinguishing characteristic of monopolar electrosurgery is its wide range of tissue effects obtainable with just minor variations in technique. For instance, the energy can be "applied" without making tissue contact (yielding the superficial desiccation of *fulguration* outlined in the former chapter). Noncontact desiccation is not possible with either bipolar devices or ultrasonic energy. Varying effects are then possible depending on which portion (size) of the electrode is applied to the tissue. Given the same wattage, application of an edge to tissue under tension might provide both a desiccating and cutting effect; the flat surface of the same electrode provides a desiccating effect which is then further enhanced by coapting the tissue in the jaws of an articulating electrode. Finally, the mechanical effects of shears and conventional dissecting instruments can be supplemented with thermal energy with the tap of a toe or finger. (To be certain, the author recognizes the superior macrodesiccating effects of enhanced bipolar and ultrasonic devices on larger vessels and greater thicknesses of tissue. The surgical benefits of monopolar are related to meticulous dissection of adventitial tissue and peritoneum around vital structures).

An Electrosurgical Alert for Single Port Laparoscopy

Single port laparoscopy offers potential cosmetic benefit but also raises electrosurgical concerns due to two considerations. First, the constraints imposed by single port technology substantially increase the actual size of zone 2 (Fig. 4.4a, b and c) where instruments are neither within the view of the laparoscope nor inside of the cannula and may be in contact with bowel or other viscera. Second, surgical instruments and the laparoscope are in much closer proximity than with traditional operations. Figure 4.4a outlines the ideal separation of instruments but the reality Fig. 4.4b is close proximity of active instruments. The potential for thermal injury due to stray currents of insulation failure, capacitive coupling, and direct coupling is substantially increased. Figure 4.4c shows the four zones of the elecrtical path of a typical laparoscopic instrument introduced through a trocar. Zones 2 and 3 are out of the Surgeon's field of view.

The most important component of safety is awareness of and reaction to the potential risk. The increased "single port" risk for injury from capacitive coupling as well as direct coupling to the laparoscope would be lessened if the port were electrically conductive and not an insulator (an insulating port limits dispersion of any stray current to biologic tissue). Defects in the insulation are difficult to visualize and may deliver 100% of the intended current to nontarget tissue; monitoring of the integrity of the active electrodes has been recommended. Alternate energy sources may be used, but they offer less utility and greater expense.

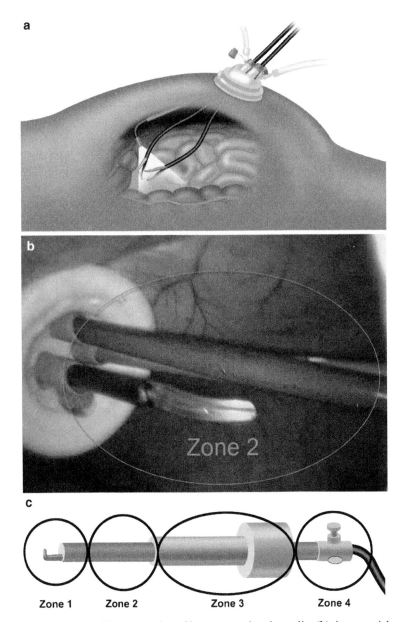

Fig. 4.4. (**a**) The ideal separation of instruments, but the reality (**b**) the potential for stray current to be recognized and to cause injury depends on the location (zone) on the instrument (**c**) is close proximity of active instruments.

The Argon Beam Enhanced Fulguration

As outlined in the previous chapter regarding argon beam enhancement, the argon gas provides an electron rich media that transmits electrical current effectively to tissue. Further, the sprayed gas blows blood from the tissue surface, thus creating a clear current-tissue interface and facilitating a superficial thermal change of fulguration. Enhanced argon beam application has its greatest theoretical value with raw irregular surfaces with capillary oozing as might occur with liver transection. However, there are potential life-threatening risks to the use of the argon beam. First, the instillation of the gas into a closed compartment (i.e., during laparoscopy) can increase intra-abdominal pressure, perhaps to the point of compartment syndrome. If the device is being used, the surgeon and anesthesiologist should monitor intra-abdominal pressure. The surgeon should use the lowest effective flow rate of the argon gas and leave a port open to allow egress of the gas. Second, the tip of the argon-enhanced electrode should be well away from the tissue to reduce the risk of direct instillation of argon gas into an open vein and subsequent gas embolism. Finally, one should be wary of using the device during hypotension or patient instability (related to hemorrhage) as the aforementioned complications manifest themselves with further hypotension and instability.

Conclusion

It is not a novel idea that a surgeon should possess an elementary understanding of the biophysics and risks of any energy source. There is a far stretch from minimal understanding to mastery of application. Hopefully, this discourse provides basic elementary material but more so poses the challenge to the gifted surgeon who recognizes, appreciates, and desires to improve the art form of our daily work. Full exploitation of the energy source will only be achieved through appreciation of the art of the science and the science of the art.

No one is an artist unless he carries his picture in his head before painting it, and is sure of his method and composition.

Claude Monet

Monet's work is an appropriate analogy for the advancing surgeon. At the risk of over simplification, Monet painted reflections of light and not objects. Thus, his genuine advancement came through his unique focus on light and his ability to transfer the cerebral image to canvas. The challenge was for the mind, the eye, and the hand. In a similar fashion, the gifted electrosurgeon studies current (which cannot be seen) and paints its reflections of thermal change. The mastery occurs first in the mind.

References

1. Cushing H, Bovie WT. Electrosurgery as an aid to the removal of intracranial tumors. Surg Gynecol Obstet. 1928;47:751–85.
2. Kelly HA, Ward GE. Electrosurgery. Philadelphia: W. B. Saunders; 1932. p. 1–9.
3. Voyles C, Tucker R. Education and engineering solutions for potential problems with laparoscopic monopolar electrosurgery. Am J Surg. 1992;164:57–62.
4. Veyckemans F, Michel I. Venous gas embolism from an argon coagulator. Anesthesiology. 1996;85(2):443–5.
5. ECRI. Fatal gas embolism caused by overpressurization during laparoscopic use of argon enhanced coagulation. Health Devices. 1994;23(6):257–9.

5. Bipolar Electrosurgical Devices

Chan W. Park and Dana D. Portenier

Bleeding is an inevitable result of surgery, and throughout history, there has always been a need for efficient and effective methods of achieving hemostasis during surgery. The use of heat to cauterize tissues and to control hemorrhage began in prehistory, long before the era of modern surgery. The application of heat to human tissues results in the denaturation of proteins and cellular/structural changes within the vasculature. However, the direct delivery of heat to cauterize tissues was limited to superficial sites and was, at best, cumbersome to perform until the development of radiofrequency (RF) electrosurgery.

As described previously (see Chap. 2), RF electrosurgical devices achieve hemostasis through the ionic conversion of high frequency electromagnetic energy to mechanical energy and then to thermal energy within the target tissue. Monopolar instruments that deliver RF electrical energy via a single active electrode were first introduced in the late nineteenth century [1], and have enabled remarkable surgical results. Able to desiccate, coagulate, vaporize, cut, and fulgurate tissues, monopolar surgical devices are at the top of any surgical instrument card today. However, these devices are not without limitations. By design, monopolar devices require the placement of a dispersive electrode at a remote site on the patient's body, and this poses a significant risk for remote/collateral injury and requires usage of greater voltage, further increasing the extent of potential harm. In addition, the lack of precision and control of many monopolar RF electrosurgical instruments limits surgical effectiveness in electricity-sensitive tissues, in intricate surgical procedures, and in "wet" surgical fields contaminated by blood and other fluids. In order to overcome these limitations of monopolar instruments, bipolar electrosurgical devices were first developed in the early twentieth century [2].

By utilizing two active electrodes that can more precisely control (and limit) the flow of electrical current through only the targeted (or "grasped") tissue area, bipolar instruments greatly reduced the risk of collateral/remote injury and the amount of voltage necessary to achieve the desired

L.S. Feldman et al. (eds.), *The SAGES Manual on the Fundamental
Use of Surgical Energy (FUSE)*, DOI 10.1007/978-1-4614-2074-3_5,
© Springer Science+Business Media, LLC 2012

tissue effect. More recent advances in surgical technology and the growth of minimally invasive surgery (MIS) have enabled the development of increasingly compact and efficient bipolar devices that are able to achieve optimal tissue effects in a wide variety of clinical applications while minimizing overall surgical risk. This chapter discusses the fundamentals of bipolar electrosurgical instrument design and presents a brief review of current bipolar technology and literature with an emphasis on surgical efficacy and safety.

Bipolar Technology: Device Design and Mechanisms

There are a wide variety of electrosurgical devices available in today's high-tech surgical environment. As described in Chap. 2 all contemporary electrosurgery is "bipolar" as it requires two electrodes - an active electrode and a second electrode for completion of the electrical circuit. However, based on the location of these two electrodes, RF electrosurgical devices can be categorized as being either monopolar or bipolar (Fig. 5.1). The primary difference is that bipolar instruments allow the application of both electrodes on the target tissue thereby

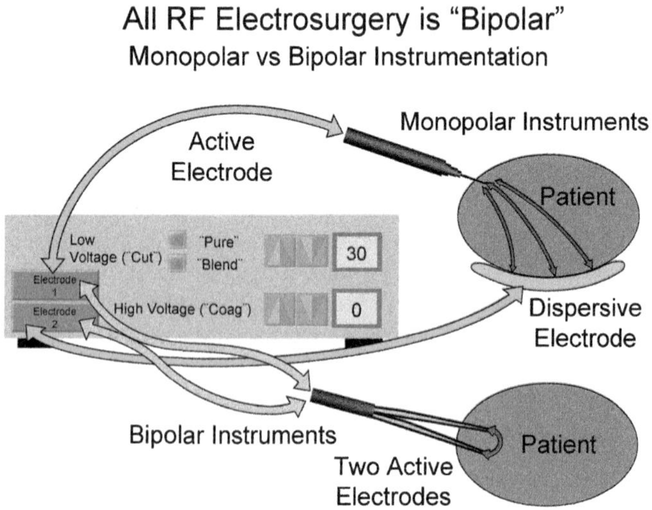

Fig. 5.1. Mono- and bipolar electrosurgery.

limiting the passage of current through only the desired area and removing the remainder of the patient's body from the electrosurgical "circuit." Furthermore, bipolar instruments can be designed so that both of the electrodes are "active" whereas with monopolar devices, the second electrode is placed on the patient remote from the surgical field, and is designed to disperse the electrical current, preventing the elevation of temperature in adjacent tissue and the creation of an electrosurgical effect.

Bipolar devices achieve tissue sealing and hemostasis by two primary mechanisms: compression of tissue and the local delivery of RF energy that results in cellular and tissue heating. First, the direct compression of a bleeding vessel obstructs the continued flow of blood promoting the development of a proximal thrombus and eliminating "heat sink" (continued flow of blood cools the tissues and interferes with coagulation). However, improper or overcompression of the tissue may result in electrical bypass and ineffective sealing of the target tissue (Fig. 5.2). Next, as described in Chap. 2, the delivery of RF energy to a target vessel produces heat and restructures the protein matrix of the vascular wall resulting in the formation of a hemostatic seal. The presence of water and ions within the tissue enables the ionic oscillation and ultimate conversion of RF energy into intracellular heat, and as the tissue temperature rises, different surgical effects such as coagulation, desiccation, and vaporization may occur.

However, while increasing electrosurgical precision and safety, bipolar instruments can affect only a relatively small amount of tissue at a time, which limits its efficacy as a rapid tissue-cutting instrument. Bipolar instruments were initially designed to produce coagulation and for sealing vessels in intricate surgical fields. In fact, some of the earliest

Electrodes touch and bypass tissue

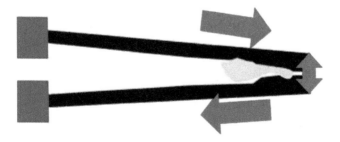

Fig. 5.2. Electrical bypass due to overcompression.

bipolar instruments were fine forceps utilized in intricate neurosurgical procedures [2]. Since these devices, designed specifically to disperse energy over a larger electrode surface area, were not intended to produce significant tissue vaporization, they were relatively ineffective for cutting through tissues. Electrosurgical cutting requires the delivery of enough energy to elevate intracellular temperature to 100°C or more, which results in the rapid conversion of water to steam. This, in turn, creates a massive volumetric expansion of the intracellular contents, and together with the thermally induced impact on the cell wall results in cellular vaporization. Vaporization requires focused delivery of RF energy using electrodes with a very small surface area, such as a blade or needle tip. Electrosurgical coagulation or vessel sealing is best achieved by avoiding the complete destruction of tissue, and today, most proprietary bipolar electrosurgical units (ESUs) will attempt to deliver only enough energy to raise the target tissue temperature above the threshold for protein bond to degradation (approximately 60°C). Furthermore, the electrosurgical energy is delivered in an interrupted fashion (the ESU rapidly cycles "on and off") to allow for tissue cooling and reduce lateral thermal spread.

Traditional ESUs were not designed to deliver pulsed outputs to reduce lateral thermal spread and lacked impedance or temperature feedback mechanisms to limit the delivery of energy to target tissues. This inefficient system of energy delivery was controlled manually by the operating surgeon based on visual cues (e.g., tissue color changes, smoke production, etc.) and this often resulted in premature cutting of tissues before coagulation was complete. This was due, in part, to the fundamental bipolar design of the hand piece which allowed both jaws of the device to be active. As energy was delivered from both jaws to a target vessel from the outside in, the superficial tissues became desiccated and visibly change color even before the core tissues reached denaturation states sufficient for hemostasis. Conversely, since electrical current follows the path of least resistance, unabated application of energy to a target vessel increased the electrical resistance (impedance) due to the loss of water content (desiccation) and resulted in the preferential flow of current through less resistive, surrounding tissues (Fig. 5.3). This "mushroom effect" extended the risk of collateral damage beyond lateral thermal spread. Thus, surgeons were forced to face the challenge of "estimating" the correct timing of when to stop energy delivery.

Modern ESUs and proprietary bipolar vessel sealing devices incorporate sophisticated microprocessors and feedback systems that monitor impedance (resistance) and/or temperature and automatically adjust the delivery of RF electrical energy in order to ensure adequate

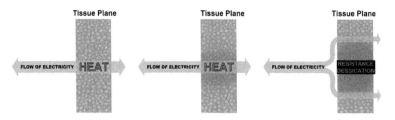

Fig. 5.3. Mushroom effect: unabated application of energy increases collateral injury.

tissue sealing while minimizing collateral tissue damage. These feedback mechanisms maximize the benefits of bipolar electrosurgical devices providing consistent vessel sealing (up to a maximum vessel diameter of 7 mm) while limiting the extent of collateral tissue injury and enhancing operative efficiency through less formation of smoke and carbonization. Referred to as "smart generators" of electrosurgical energy, modern ESUs for bipolar vessel sealing instruments accomplish these rapid adjustments in near real-time and even provide audible signals to indicate when adequate coagulation has been achieved.

With the recent growth of minimally invasive surgery (MIS), there has been an increasing need for compact bipolar devices that can do more than just safely seal bleeding vessels. Most bipolar surgical devices incorporate proprietary modifications to the basic mechanism of bipolar instrument design and deliver the ability to seal and even cut target tissues without compromising patient safety and hemostatic efficacy. Some devices incorporate a cutting blade (built into the center of the jaw) and others maximize ESU energy delivery through specialized instrument jaw designs to achieve bipolar vessel sealing and electrosurgical cutting simultaneously and/or sequentially. Taking surgical efficiency one step further, innovative bipolar device designs such as a dual action jaw that allows mechanical tissue dissection, bipolar instruments with built-in monopolar electrosurgical dissection tips, and laparoscopic bipolar devices that are able to grasp and manipulate intra-abdominal organs with greater stability and minimal tissue trauma all contribute to shorter operating times through minimization of instrument exchanges. Contemporary bipolar devices enhance surgical efficiency and are able to rapidly achieve consistent vessel sealing within seconds (with seal bursting pressures significantly above physiologic blood pressure levels [3–5]).

Currently Available Bipolar Electrosurgical Devices

It is beyond the scope of this chapter to provide a comprehensive overview of contemporary bipolar technology and highlight the key differences in instrument designs. However, it is important to note that there are other devices such as ultrasonic dissectors and thermal tissue sealing devices that are similar in appearance to bipolar electrosurgical devices and are able to seal and divide tissues. Those devices are neither bipolar nor monopolar electrosurgical instruments. While in-depth discussion is beyond the scope of this chapter, briefly, ultrasonic devices (discussed in Chap. 7) utilize rapid conversion of electrical energy into mechanical energy to induce frictional heating, sealing, and vaporization of target tissues. Likewise, newer thermal tissue sealing devices use direct application of heat (cautery), *without* the conduction of electrical energy through target tissues to achieve hemostasis, tissue sealing, and division. By contrast, electrosurgical devices conduct electrical current through tissues and are fundamentally distinct from ultrasonic dissectors and thermal tissue sealing devices.

Select Review of Literature

Several studies have compared the vessel sealing characteristics of different types of bipolar electrosurgical devices. Lamberton and associates tested 5-mm bipolar (Ligasure V, Gyrus PK, and Enseal) and ultrasonic dissector (Harmonic Scapel ACE™) devices in a bovine (arterial vessel explant) model [3]. End points included burst pressure and vessel sealing time, measurements of lateral thermal spread outside of target tissues, and both subjective and objective assessments of smoke production and resultant changes in surgical visibility in a simulated laparoscopic environment. Each device was tested repeatedly on 5-mm diameter vessels: 20 applications per device for assessment of seal time, and 10 applications per device for lateral thermal spread, burst pressure, and objective visibility measurements. Smoke production and visibility were objectively quantified by measurement of particulates using a laser photometer at a distance of 5 cm from the target tissue (the highest values during vessel sealing were recorded) and subjective scores of visibility were obtained from blinded video review by ten independent evaluators.

All devices achieved burst pressures above physiologic blood pressure; however, there was a significant degree of variability within and across devices. The Ligasure device attained consistent seals with burst pressure above 150 mmHg for a majority (80%) of repeated applications; all other devices performed at 50%. The amount of time needed for vessel sealing (and cutting) was also shortest for the Ligasure device and longest for the EnSeal, but all devices achieved results within a matter of seconds (range 10–19 s). Maximum lateral tissue temperature (measured by needle thermistor placed 2 mm from edge) was lowest for the ultrasonic device (49.9°C) and this difference was statistically significant when compared to the Gyrus PK (64.5°C), but there were no statistically significant differences between the ultrasonic device and the Ligasure (55.5°C) and EnSeal (58.9°C) lateral thermal measurements. Finally, the ultrasonic device produced the least amount of particulates/smoke (2.9 ppm) and the Ligasure (12.5 ppm) and EnSeal (23.6 ppm) devices produced slightly greater amounts, but the Gyrus PK device (74.1 ppm) produced significantly higher levels. Subjective ratings of visibility were consistent with the objective measurements of particulate/smoke production.

In another study comparing safety and efficacy of four devices (Harmonic scalpel ACE, Ligasure V, Ligasure Atlas, and EnSeal) by Person, et al., blood vessels of varying types and sizes were harvested utilizing the different devices [4]. Vessel diameters, speed of vessel sealing, and burst pressures of sealed vessels were studied (Fig. 5.4). The EnSeal

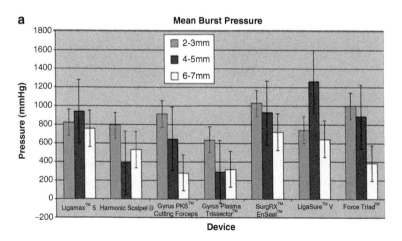

Fig. 5.4. (**a–c**) Summary of evaluated parameters and histopathology findings. (From Person et al. [4], with kind permission of Springer Science+Business Media).

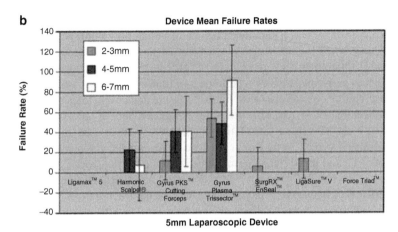

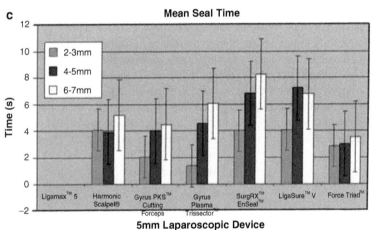

Fig. 5.4. (continued)

device created seals with the highest mean burst pressure (678 mmHg), but all devices achieved seals with mean burst pressures well above physiologic blood pressure levels (Ligasure V—380 mmHg, Ligasure Atlas 489 mmHg, Harmonic ACE—435 mmHg). Interestingly, histologic evaluations of vascular seals were undertaken, but heterogeneity of results and a small sample size precluded definitive conclusions. Nevertheless, the Harmonic ACE and EnSeal devices achieved the narrowest seal widths, and although the EnSeal caused less denaturation of adventitial collagen in vessels, it was associated with greater wall injury to proximal inner wall layers.

Recently, Newcomb and colleagues compared a variety of 5-mm laparoscopic tissue sealing devices on a porcine (arterial explant) model to assess for device-specific safety and efficacy [5]. Vessel burst pressures and seal failure rates along with length of time for vessel sealing were utilized as comparative end points. Multiple bipolar devices (Gyrus PKS cutting forceps, Gyrus Plasma Trissector, Ethicon EnSeal, Covidien Ligasure V), an ultrasonic tissue sealing device (Harmonic Scalpel), and a mechanical clip applier (Ligamax 5) were among the surgical instruments studied. All devices achieved supra-physiologic mean burst pressures (range of 285–1,261 mmHg) when results were averaged across all vessels sizes (2–7 mm in diameter); however, seal failure rates were noted to be highly variable (Tables 5.1 and 5.2). The ultrasonic device and the Gyrus bipolar devices were noted to have the highest mean failure rates 7–22% and 12–92%, respectively. All devices achieved vessel seals within seconds (<8 s maximum), and increasing diameters of vessels required longer seal times across all devices. Of note, seal time was not recorded for the mechanical clip applier. The authors concluded that while the lowest failure rates and highest burst pressures were achieved with both the EnSeal and Ligasure devices, there was a shorter seal time with the Ligasure device.

Other reports on bipolar instruments present data that are consistent with the studies summarized above; however, there is wide variability across study designs. Thus, it is somewhat difficult to draw meaningful conclusions of device superiority (or inferiority) from available data [6–12]. While the current volume of literature demonstrates the significant achievements of surgical innovation and the ongoing technological evolution of electrosurgical instruments, the plethora of commercially available products in today's surgical environment, ongoing development of newer products, and the rapid turnover and continued modifications of

Table 5.1. Summary of the evaluated parameters comparing blood vessel sealing devices.

Instrument	No. of specimens	Vessel diameter (mm)	Quality of seal#	Speed of seal (s)	Burst pressure (mmHg)
EnSeal™	50	4.1 ± 1.5	3.98	4.1 ± 0.9	678 ± 184+
LigaSure™ V	55	3.8 ± 1.6	3.93	5.2 ± 2.1	380 ± 135
LigaSure Atlas™	27	4.8 ± 0.6*	3.78	7.9 ± 2.2	489 ± 270
Harmonic ACE™	52	3.3 ± 1.0*	4	3.3 ± 1.0	435 ± 321

From Newcomb et al. [5], with kind permission of Springer Science + Business Media
*P=0.0006; #P=NS; +P<0.0001

Table 5.2. Histopathology findings comparing blood vessel sealing devices.

Instrument	Seal width (mm) (mean (range))	Denatured adventitial collagen (mm) (mean (range))	Wall layer dissection (%)	Gas formation (%)	Blood pockets (%)	Proximal wall injury
EnSeal™	1.0 (0.1–2.4)	0.1 (0.0–0.6)	60	60	40	4/5
LigaSure™ V	1.8 (0.5–3.4)	0.4 (0.0–1.4)	100	75	25	3/4
LigaSure Atlas™	2.5 (1.6–3.7)	1.5 (0.5–2.8)	75	75	25	1/3[a]
Harmonic ACE™	0.9 (0.6–1.4)	1.0 (0.1–2.0)	50	100	0	3/4

From Newcomb et al. [5], with kind permission of Springer Science + Business Media

%, the percentage of the specimens in which each finding was observed

[a] One specimen had insufficient tissue proximal to the seal

existing instrument designs make comparative studies difficult to conduct and confound comparative analysis. This highlights the importance of improving the surgeon's understanding of the principles of RF electrosurgery and the critical need for the surgeon's ability to evaluate the many devices, their design and proprietary claims of instrument capabilities. Lastly, the true measures of a device's safety and efficacy remain as yet undefined. While bursting pressures, vessel sealing times, and seal histology help to quantify an instrument's capabilities, what specific characteristics of a device's form and function yield truly relevant clinical benefits still remain unanswered. Nevertheless, it is not difficult to agree that, when used properly, bipolar electrosurgical devices have established favorable operating safety profiles and are capable of consistently achieving hemostatic tissue seals in vessels up to 7 mm in diameter.

Best Practices for Safety

The following section outlines recommendations for proper bipolar RF electrosurgical instrument use and some best practices to enhance safety.

Contact with Tissues

Bipolar devices require proper contact between the jaw surface and the target tissue in order to achieve adequate vessel apposition, coagulation, and sealing. Excessive tension or grasping too much tissue in a single "bite" will hinder tissue apposition and may jeopardize coagulation. Additionally, charring or build-up of coagulum on the device surface, which inhibits device–tissue interface, must be avoided and promptly addressed by frequent cleansing with a damp cloth. As mentioned previously, desiccated tissues will increase impedance between the jaws and potentially increase the risk of collateral damage and lateral thermal injury.

Adherence to Tissues

Occasionally, a bipolar device may become "stuck" or adherent to the target tissue. Care must be taken to minimize traumatic detachment, and the use of mechanical force is discouraged as this may cause disruption of the newly created vessel seal. Reactivation of the bipolar device under irrigation will create steam bubbles that may help to dislodge the tissue. An alternative is to reactivate the bipolar device with minimal jaw apposition (to "reheat" the protein bonds at the tissue–device interface).

Overlapping a Seal

Although modern bipolar devices have feedback systems that ensure adequate tissue sealing and obviate the need for manual control of energy delivery, sometimes it is desirable to overlap vessel seals. This should be considered especially in areas with anatomical tension and in areas where there may be significant consequences from vessel seal disruption. When overlapping seals, ~30–50% of the existing seal should be overlapped by the device jaw, and fresh unsealed tissue should never be left in between two seals.

Grasping Materials Other than Tissue

Although the bipolar design limits the flow of current between the jaws of the device, activation in very close proximity to highly conductive materials (e.g., metal clips, staples, etc.) may cause unpredictable current migration and injury. Furthermore, the bipolar device should not be used to seal or cut tissue contained within a staple line or clip, and bipolar devices with mechanical blades should never be used to cut sutures or materials that may dull the sharpness of the blade.

Lateral Thermal Spread

There is a risk of lateral thermal spread up to several millimeters. It is always clinically prudent to leave a margin for safety when utilizing any electrosurgical device and the surgeon should avoid activation in close contact with surrounding critical structures.

Patients with Comorbid Conditions

Patients with comorbid conditions such as liver cirrhosis, chronic steroid use, atherosclerosis, malnutrition, diabetes, collagen vascular disorder, systemic infections, etc. may exhibit differences in tissue composition, structure, and morphology that may alter or inhibit the function and efficacy of a bipolar device. Caution must be taken in these situations and alternative surgical methods may be required.

Conclusions

From the early days of direct cautery and monopolar RF instrumentation, bipolar electrosurgical devices have evolved and enabled remarkable surgical outcomes in today's technologically advanced operating room. Inherent in the bipolar design is an increased degree of electrosurgical safety, and through ongoing innovation, these instruments continue to enhance surgical efficacy and efficiency. Currently, a large variety of electrosurgical devices exist, each with its own unique characteristics and features, but comparative studies that allow meaningful analyses and evaluation are somewhat lacking. Further research is necessary and mandatory in order to keep pace with the rapid advancements in this field.

References

1. Massarweh NN, Cosgriff NN, Slakey DP. Electrosurgery: history, principles, and current and future uses. J Am Coll Surg. 2006;202:520–30.
2. Malis LI. Electrosurgery and bipolar technology. Neurosurgery. 2006;58(Suppl 1): ONS 1–12.
3. Lamberton GR, Hsi RS, Jin DH, et al. Prospective comparison of four laparoscopic vessel ligation devices. J Endourol. 2008;22:2307–12.
4. Person B, Vivas DA, Ruiz D, Talcott M, Coad JE, Wexner SD. Comparison of four energy-based vascular sealing and cutting instruments: a porcine model. Surg Endosc. 2008;22:534–8.
5. Newcomb WL, Hope WW, Schmeizer TM, et al. Comparison of blood vessel sealing among new electrosurgical and ultrasonic devices. Surg Endosc. 2009;23:90–6.
6. Sutton PA, Awad S, Perkins AC, Lobo DN. Comparison of lateral thermal spread using monopolar and bipolar diathermy, the harmonic scalpel and the ligasure. Br J Surg. 2010;97:428–33.
7. Targarona EM, Balague C, Marin J, et al. Energy sources of laparoscopic colectomy: a prospective randomized comparison of conventional electrosurgery, bipolar compter-controlled electrosurgery and ultrasonic dissection. Operative outcome and costs analysis. Surg Innov. 2005;12(4):339–44.

8. Katsuno G, Nagakari K, Fukunaga M. Comparison of two different energy-based vascular sealing systems for the hemostasis of various types of arteries: a porcine model-evaluation of LigaSure ForceTriad™. J Laparoendosc Adv Surg Tech A. 2010;20(9):747–51.

9. Song C, Tang B, Campbell PA, Cuschieri A. Thermal spread and heat absorbance differences between open and laparoscopic surgeries during energized dissections by electrosurgical instruments. Surg Endosc. 2009;23(11):2480–7.

10. Lakeman M, Kruitwagen RF, Vos MC, Roovers JP. Electrosurgical bipolar vessel sealing versus conventional clamping and suturing for total abdominal hysterectomy: a randomized trial. J Minim Invasive Gynecol. 2008;15(5):547–53.

11. Levy B, Emery L. Randomized trial of suture versus electrosurgical bipolar vessel sealing in vaginal hysterectomy. Obstet Gynecol. 2003;102(1):147–51.

12. Macario A, Dexter F, Sypal J, Cosgriff N, Heniford BT. Operative time and other outcomes of the electrothermal bipolar vessel sealing system (LigaSure) versus other methods for surgical hemostasis: a meta-analysis. Surg Innov. 2008;15(4):284–91.

6. Electrosurgical Energy in Gastrointestinal Endoscopy

Brian J. Dunkin and Calvin D. Lyons

The safe use of radiofrequency (RF) electrosurgery within the lumen of the gastrointestinal (GI) tract requires knowledge of the unique aspects of this environment. This chapter will describe common devices used for cutting, coagulation, and ablation in GI endoscopy, give practical recommendations for their use, and provide safety tips to avoid complications. The principles of RF electrosurgery and an understanding of its interaction with implantable cardiac devices, which serves as the basis for all electrosurgical procedures, are covered elsewhere in this book.

Hardware

As in surgery, electrosurgical devices in GI endoscopy can be categorized into groups based on the design of the instrumentation.

Monopolar Devices

Monopolar instrumentation can be used to resect, cut, or coagulate mucosal lesions as well as for protein coagulation which results in collagen contraction and tightening of a sphincter. The most common monopolar device used for resection is the polypectomy snare (Fig. 6.1a). Such instruments are available in a variety of diameters, thicknesses, and configurations requiring the endoscopist to choose the appropriate size and configuration to successfully resect the polyp while avoiding damage to surrounding tissue. Monopolar biopsy forceps are also available ("hot biopsy" forceps, Fig. 6.1b) and are used to resect small polyps while ablating surrounding adenomatous tissue. The most aggressive mucosal

L.S. Feldman et al. (eds.), *The SAGES Manual on the Fundamental Use of Surgical Energy (FUSE)*, DOI 10.1007/978-1-4614-2074-3_6, © Springer Science+Business Media, LLC 2012

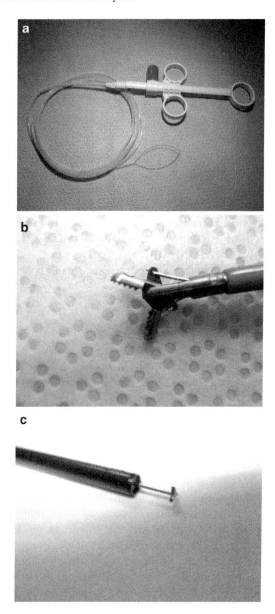

Fig. 6.1. (**a**) Polypectomy snare. (**b**) Hot biopsy forceps. (**c**) Endoscopic submucosal dissection (ESD) knife.

resections in the GI tract are achieved with endoscopic submucosal dissection (ESD). This technique enables full thickness mucosal resection down to the muscularis propria using monopolar ESD knives that allow for the achievement of en bloc resections many centimeters in size (Fig. 6.1c).

The most common monopolar cutting device is the monopolar sphincterotome used during endoscopic retrograde cholangiopancreatography (ERCP). A Pull Sphincterotome consists of a bowing wire electrode mounted on the end of a flexible catheter (Fig. 6.2a) that can be attached to an electrosurgical generator or unit (ESU). The wire is positioned within the papilla of Vater so that it traverses the sphincter of Oddi and is used to cut the sphincter when the ESU is activated (Fig. 6.2b). The cut widens the opening of the papilla so that larger instrumentation can be introduced into the bile and pancreatic ducts or for the extraction of stones. An electrosurgical Needle Knife Spincterotome enables the endoscopist to perform a "freehand" sphincterotomy when a pull sphincterotome cannot be introduced into the papilla. A fine wire electrode for division of the sphincter protrudes from the end of a plastic catheter (Fig. 6.2c). Even in experienced hands, this device is associated with a higher complication rate and must be used with care.

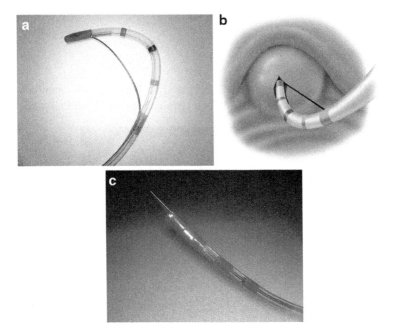

Fig. 6.2. (**a**) Pull Sphincterotome. (**b**) The pull sphincterotome is positioned in the papilla of Vater which is cut with the application of current. (**c**) Needle Knife Spincterotome.

As described in previous chapters, argon gas can facilitate arcing of electrical current between the electrode and the tissue and is usually used in conjunction with high-voltage modulated waveforms. This noncontact method of fulguration, called argon plasma coagulation (APC), is particularly effective in managing superficial mucosal lesions such as arteriovenous malformations (AVMs) and radiation proctitis. Using APC, the mucosa can be fulgurated in a "painting" fashion to treat larger areas without deep penetration of the tissue or disruption of the resultant coagulum (Fig. 6.3). Flexible endoscopic APC probes come in three configurations—forward, side, and radial fire.

A special device not commonly thought of in the group of monopolar instruments is the Stretta® catheter (Fig. 6.4). This balloon-based radial electrode array is used to apply RF energy to the muscularis propria of the lower esophagus resulting in collagen contraction, tissue thickening, and ablation of local innervation which leads to a more effective lower esophageal sphincter in patients suffering from gastroesophageal reflux disease. The device has continuous temperature and impedance sensing at the electrode tips and a perfusion system to cool the overlying mucosa. The dispersive electrode is placed between the shoulder blades on the back to assure the shortest path of conductivity.

Bipolar Devices

There are only two bipolar RF electrosurgical instruments commonly used in GI endoscopy—the multipolar electrocoagulation (MPEC) probe

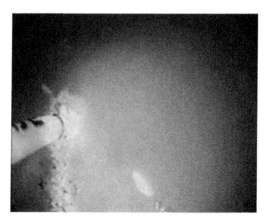

Fig. 6.3. Argon plasma coagulation (APC).

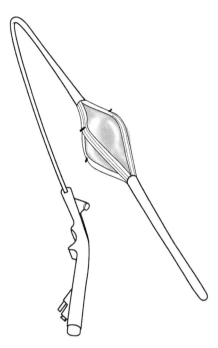

Fig. 6.4. Balloon-based radial electrode array (Stretta® catheter).

(Fig. 6.5a) and the radiofrequency array for ablation of esophageal mucosa (Fig. 6.5b). The MPEC has a gold electrode wrapped around the tip of a flexible 7 or 10 French catheter. It is used to coagulate bleeding lesions in the GI tract or to desiccate superficial lesions of the mucosa. It may have an integrated injection needle for delivering a sclerosant and an irrigation channel to clear blood and clot away from the targeted lesion. Because of the gold-colored electrode at the tip of the MPEC, it is often called a "gold" probe.

The radiofrequency (RF) array ablation catheters are newer bipolar devices used to ablate the mucosa of the GI tract. They are most commonly used to destroy intestinal metaplasia in the esophagus, but have also been used to ablate mucosa in other areas of the GI tract as well as manage bleeding from AVMs and radiation proctitis. There are two configurations—a balloon-based array that ablates a circumferential area of esophageal mucosa 3 cm long and a paddle electrode for directed ablation therapy. In both devices, tightly spaced electrodes conduct high-voltage RF electrical energy for short intervals to superficially ablate the GI mucosa down to, but not through, the muscularis mucosa. The

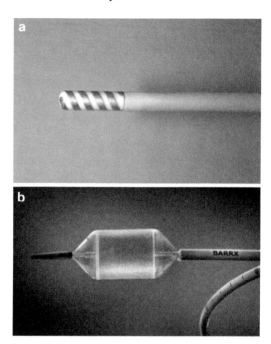

Fig. 6.5. (**a**) Multipolar electrocoagulation (MPEC) probe. (**b**) Balloon based array RF ablation catheter. (Courtesy of BARRX, Sunnyvale, CA, USA. Used by permission. The use of any BARRX photo or image does not imply BARRX review or endorsement of any article or publication).

circumferential catheter also senses impedance and will disarm if contact is lost with the mucosa. RF ablation of dysplastic intestinal metaplasia in the esophagus has transformed the management of this disease and enabled many patients to avoid surgery.

Other

There is one other device commonly used in flexible GI endoscopy to manage bleeding. It is a flexible Teflon-tipped catheter that delivers energy to the targeted tissue by direct heat transfer (cautery). When activated this "heater probe" simply is heated and this thermal energy is transferred to the tissue via direct contact. The heater probe is not an electrosurgical device, but often misclassified as one by the novice endoscopist.

Patient Preparation

It is as important to prepare a patient properly for a flexible GI procedure as for a surgical one. However, since many endoscopy centers operate "open units" where patients may come for a screening colonoscopy without a prior physician office visit, the endoscopist must rapidly assess the patient for risk of potential complications from electrosurgical energy. Particular attention must be paid to the presence of body jewelry and rhythm management devices (see Chaps. 3 and 12). For monopolar instrumentation, placement of the dispersive electrode must also be done with care to ensure proper contact and to avoid exposing it to fluid during the procedure. In addition, it is important that the patient has had adequate bowel preparation. For upper endoscopy, this usually means no solid food within 8–12 h of the procedure and no liquids for at least four prior. For colonoscopy, bowel preparation is even more critical to minimize the presence of methane gas, which can cause an explosion. Mannitol bowel preparations in particular are avoided because of their association with methane gas build up.

Principles of RF Electrosurgery in Gastrointestinal Endoscopy

The most feared complications of GI endoscopy are perforation and bleeding. Care must be taken to correctly apply electrosurgical energy in the GI tract at the proper device settings to avoid these complications. It is particularly important to recognize that the thickness of the muscular layer of the GI tract varies considerably from location to location. The stomach and rectum are among the thickest structures, while the duodenum and right colon are among the thinnest. Energy application must be varied by site to avoid full thickness injury.

It is also important to understand the principles of current density (see Chaps. 2 and 3) when excising lesions in the GI tract. During polypectomy the current density is highest where the snare is tightened around the base of the polyp (Fig. 6.6). Therefore, the larger the base of the polyp, or the wider the snare, the more energy required to section it. Too much energy may result in full thickness thermal injury and possible perforation.

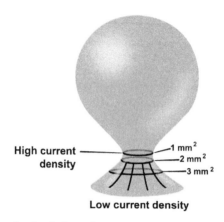

High current
density
- 1 mm^2
- 2 mm^2
- 3 mm^2

Low current density

Fig. 6.6. Current density during polypectomy.

Current density is also important when performing an endoscopic sphincterotomy (ES) during ERCP. Ideally, the pull sphincterotome is positioned into the papilla of Vater and across the area of the sphincter of Oddi using as little length of wire as possible. This will ensure more efficient delivery of energy to the target tissue while minimizing collateral thermal spread—a phenomenon that increases the risk of pancreatitis or perforation. Applying light pressure only with the cutting wire also ensures high current density at the target.

A common technique used to buffer the muscularis propria from thermal energy created in the overlying mucosa is to perform a "saline lift." An injection needle is used to pierce the mucosa and deliver saline into the potential space between the mucosal layer and the muscularis thereby creating a protective saline "bleb" that protects the muscularis from thermal damage or perforation. Saline lift polypectomy is a common technique used to remove large, flat mucosal lesions in the colon.

Bleeding ulcers in the upper GI tract can almost always be successfully controlled with endoscopic intervention. An important technique used to achieve hemostasis is called coaptive coagulation. Bleeding from an ulcer in the GI tract is most commonly emanating from the wall of a submucosal blood vessel at the base of the ulcer. To effectively seal these vessels, the hemostasis catheter (MPEC or heater probe) is pressed firmly against the vessel to collapse (i.e., coapt) the walls (Fig. 6.7). When, in such instances, high-voltage RF energy is applied, the walls seal together

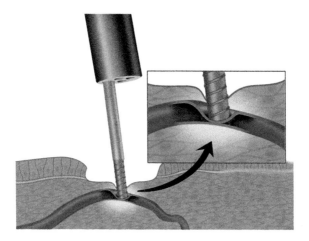

Fig. 6.7. Coaptive coagulation.

and the bleeding stops. Multiple applications of energy in the same location are recommended. In experienced hands, using a combination of injection sclerotherapy and coaptive coagulation, approximately 90% of upper GI ulcer bleeding can be controlled.

Recommended Energy Settings for Specific Procedures

Polypectomy

Bleeding from polypectomy is the most common complication occurring in up to 4% of cases. Perforation is less common at 0.5%. The smallest snare and lowest power setting to achieve the desired effect should be used. Exact power settings vary according to location in the GI tract, patient body habitus, and the amount of tissue to be divided. The waveform (output) selected should be either modulated low-voltage ("blended") or modulated high-voltage ("coagulation"). Continuous low voltage ("pure cutting current") has been shown to result in the highest postpolypectomy bleeding rates. The higher-voltage outputs ("blend" and "coag") seem to be equally effective with similar safety profiles, but the "blend" output tends to be associated with a higher risk of immediate postpolypectomy bleeding while the coag waveform is more often associated with a delayed bleed (2–8 days). Some advocate "preconditioning" pedunculated polyps by first applying "coagulation" output until the tissue blanches, followed by continuous low-voltage ("cutting") output. Use of a saline lift and tenting the mucosa at the base of the polyp are common strategies used to minimize full thickness thermal injury.

"Hot" Biopsy

This technique is used to remove diminutive polyps while ensuring that any residual tissue is ablated to minimize recurrence. A monopolar biopsy forceps grasps the sessile polyp and tents the mucosa to elevate the lesion away from the submucosa. Short bursts of "coagulation" waveform current are applied until the tissue blanches. The polyp is then excised. In principle, a tissue sample is obtained that allows correct pathologic classification of the polyp while ablating any residual adenomatous tissue. Practically, there is often thermal artifact in the specimen making pathologic interpretation difficult and the technique does not seem to consistently clear the polypectomy area of residual adenomatous tissue. There is also a significant risk for delayed bleeding. Currently, many endoscopists manage diminutive polyps by cold excision without energy using a large capacity forceps.

Bleeding Ulcers

The endoscopic management of bleeding lesions of the upper GI tract is highly successful with a large body of literature describing optimal strategies. An in-depth discussion of the topic is beyond the scope of this chapter, but a brief summary is provided in Table 6.1 with recommended MPEC energy settings and the preferred technique of application for managing the most common lesions. The successful management of UGI bleeding requires not only the correct use of RF electrosurgery, but also proper patient preparation and a multidisciplinary approach to assure best outcome.

Endoscopic Sphincterotomy

Biliary sphincterotomy is most commonly performed using a pull sphincterotome. These come with monofilament or braided wire electrodes

Table 6.1. Center for Ulcer Research and Education (CURE) MPEC settings for nonvariceal UGI hemostasis: ulcer, Dieulafoy's lesion, and Mallory–Weiss tear (without portal hypertension) treatment[a].

	Peptic ulcer			Dieulafoy's lesson		Mallory–Weiss tear
Multipolar coagulation (Gold Probe)	Active bleeding	Non-bleeding visible vessel	Adherent clot	Active bleeding	Non-bleeding visible vessel	Active bleeding
Probe size	Large	Large	Large	Large	Large	Large or small
Pressure	Very firm	Very firm	Firm	Firm	Firm	Moderate
Power setting (Watts)	12–16	12–16	12–16	12–16	12–16	12–14
Pulse duration (seconds)	10	10	10	10	10	2
End point	Bleeding stops, vessel flat and white; DUP-	Visible vessel flat and white; DUP-	NBVV or clot remnant flat and white; DUP-	Bleeding stops, vessel flat and white; DUP-	Visible vessel flat and white; DUP-	Bleeding stops, vessel flat and white; DUP-

[a]This table summarizes the guidelines for endoscopic hemostasis of nonvariceal UGI lesions for control of active bleeding or prevention of rebleeding with multipolar electrocoagulation (MPEC). The guidelines are based on randomized laboratory study results and clinical prospective studies of bleeding UGI ulcers and other nonvariceal lesions. For chronic ulcers and large lesions, large MPEC probes (e.g., 10 French) yield better hemostatic results than small probes (7 French)

of varying length and configuration. It is the endoscopist's goal to create as clean a cut as possible with the lowest chance of thermal spread, bleeding, or perforation. Monofilament wires cut more cleanly than braided designs, and, consequently, are used most commonly. Pure cutting current has the highest risk of bleeding and increased likelihood of creating an uncontrolled "zipper cut" where the energy effect is so large that an uncontrolled cut is created across the entire wall of the duodenum. To minimize bleeding and the possibility of a "zipper" cut, it is recommended to use either a blended waveform or a "pulsed" current that automatically delivers short bursts of pure cut followed by longer bursts of coagulation. Pulsed continuous currents cut more cleanly and allow for better control than blended currents.

Argon Plasma Coagulation

APC is an effective modality to achieve superficial coagulation of the GI mucosa without deeper thermal injury. It is particularly good for ablating AVMs and has been used effectively for radiation proctitis. In thin-walled areas such as the duodenum and cecum, 20 W (modulated high voltage) is usually sufficient while minimizing the risk of full thickness thermal damage. In the stomach and rectum, 40–60 W may be used. Tissue effect is also controlled by adjusting the flow rate of argon and the configuration of the APC probe (forward, side, or radial fire). Care must be taken to evacuate the argon gas intermittently throughout the procedure to prevent overdistention of the closed GI tract.

Endoscopic Submucosal Dissection

This technique is effective in removing large mucosal lesions en bloc. A saline lift is always done at the beginning of the procedure, followed by cutting through the mucosa and into the submucosal plane using an ESD knife. Standardization of energy application for ESD has not been achieved, but most practitioners use low-voltage waveforms to vaporize tissue for the dissection alternatively with modulated high-voltage waveforms as needed to stop bleeding from the fine vessels encountered in the submucosal plane.

Radiofrequency Ablation of Esophageal Mucosa

When using RF energy to ablate intestinal metaplasia (IM) in the esophagus, the required energy density and technique of application varies according to the presence of dysplasia and the chosen device. Using the balloon-based electrode array to ablate nondysplastic IM requires 10 J/cm^2 applied twice whereas dysplastic IM (low grade or high grade) requires two sequential applications of 14 J/cm^2 (Fig. 6.5b). If the RF paddle is used, 14 J/cm^2 is applied a total of four times regardless of the presence of dysplasia— two times sequentially followed by removal of the sloughed mucosa and reapplication of energy another two times. RF ablation of IM can result in esophageal strictures, but less often than with other modalities such as photodynamic therapy (PDT). RF-induced strictures are more responsive to dilation.

Safety

Performing procedures within the close lumen of the GI tract and working through the instrument channel of an endoscope present unique opportunities for complications during flexible GI endoscopy. This section provides guidance on avoidance of these complications, recognition of their occurrence, and management.

Postpolypectomy Syndrome

This complication is the result of full thickness thermal injury to the colonic wall following polypectomy. Patients usually initially feel well and are discharged from the endoscopy suite after their procedure only to return later that day or the next with abdominal pain and fever. On examination, they have localized tenderness suggesting possible colonic perforation. However, on computer tomography (CT) imaging there is no evidence of perforation. The full thickness thermal injury has resulted in localized inflammation and peritoneal irritation without perforation. These patients are managed with supportive therapy (i.e., intravenous fluids, antibiotics, and bowel rest) and monitored closely with serial examinations. Most resolve their symptoms without operative intervention. The correct application of RF electricity as described in the polypectomy section of this chapter coupled with safety adjuncts like tenting of the mucosa or saline lift during resection will help to avoid this complication.

Unintentional Direct Coupling

There are two unique scenarios in GI endoscopy that can lead to unintentional direct coupling. The first is failure to deliver the entire conductive surface of the endoscopic instrument outside of the working channel of the endoscope and into the direct view of the endoscopist. When this occurs and energy is applied, the portion of the tool that is within the working channel of the endoscope can directly couple to the tip of the scope—possibly through an insulation failure—and burn the wall of the GI tract outside of the view of the endoscopist. As a result, it is important to have the entire working area of the endoscopic device within view before applying energy.

A second unique opportunity for unintentional direct coupling occurs during removal of large pedunculated polyps. As energy is applied to the snare, the tip of the polyp may rest against the opposite wall of the colon (Fig. 6.8). This can result in unintentional delivery of energy to that site and thermal damage or perforation. To avoid this, the polyp should be rapidly moved back and forth during application of energy by "jiggling" the snare. In this way, even if there is direct coupling, it will occur for only a very brief period of time over multiple areas of the opposite wall and thus minimize significant energy delivery or thermal damage.

Incorrect Management of the Polypectomy Snare

Performing a safe polypectomy requires not only proper use of RF energy, but also of the snare itself. A unique aspect of GI endoscopy is that the devices are often "operated" by the assistant while the endoscopist targets the tissue. During snare polypectomy, it is important that the assistant not tighten the snare too quickly while the energy is

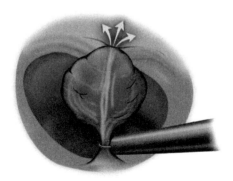

Fig. 6.8. Accidental direct coupling through a polyp to the colonic wall.

being applied. This can either result in a cold guillotine of the lesion with resultant bleeding, or embedding of the snare wire into the polyp tissue that increases the surface area in contact with the snare and decreases current density. In this "buried snare" scenario, increased levels of energy must be applied to cut through the polyp which risks full thickness thermal damage. When dealing with a buried snare, switching to the lower voltage pure cutting current may help complete the polypectomy while minimizing collateral thermal damage.

Endoscopic clips are frequently used to control bleeding or serve as a radiopaque marker. If clips have been applied near the base of a polyp, it is important to avoid placing a snare over these clips. Direct coupling between the snare and clips can result in the unintentional delivery of thermal energy to another part of the GI mucosa and possible deep thermal damage or perforation.

Conclusion

While the principles of RF electrosurgery are the same throughout the body, use of this energy in the closed environment of the GI tract results in unique scenarios that must be understood to achieve the best therapeutic results while avoiding complications. It is also important for surgeons to be familiar with common endoscopic tools so that if complications should arise, their etiology is better understood and this understanding can lead to more effective management.

References

1. Dunkin BJ, Matthes K, Jensen DM. Hemostasis (Chap. 15). In: Cohen J, editor. Successful training in gastrointestinal endoscopy. Oxford: Wiley; 2011.
2. Dunkin BJ, Joseph R. Endoluminal procedures for early gastric cancer. In: Matteoltti R, Ashley SW, editors. Minimally invasive surgical oncology. New York: Springer; 2011.
3. Rey JF, Bellenhoff U, Neumann CS, Dumonceau JM. European society of gastrointestinal endoscopy (ESGE) guideline: the use of electrosurgical units. Endoscopy. 2010;42:764–71.
4. Blocksom JM, Tokioka S, Sugawa C. Current therapy for nonvariceal upper gastrointestinal bleeding. Surg Endosc. 2004;18:186–92.

7. Ultrasonic Energy Systems

James G. Bittner IV, J. Esteban Varela, and Daniel Herron

General Principles of Ultrasonic Energy

Ultrasound refers to sound waves that have a wave frequency above the upper limit of human hearing, or greater than 20,000 Hz (20 kHz). Perhaps the best known use of ultrasound is for diagnostic imaging, where wave frequencies range from 2 to 18 megahertz (MHz). However, there is an evolving spectrum of therapeutic uses of ultrasonic energy, including the CUSA device, and surgical cutting and coagulating systems, the topic of this chapter. Such systems use a frequency of 23–55 kHz to transmit energy to surgical instruments that may be used for transection of tissue and coagulation of blood vessels. Such ultrasonic surgical devices manifest their tissue effect by one or a combination of mechanisms that include mechanical cutting, desiccation and protein coagulation, and a hybrid form of vaporization and facilitated dissection in selected tissues that is called *cavitation*. The fact that this spectrum of tissue effects can be achieved absent an electrical circuit and the inherent associated risks is attractive, but adverse events are still possible because of the heat generated in the tips of these devices. Consequently, and similar with other systems, it is critical that the surgeon understands both the basic principles and safe use of these devices.

Ultrasonic transection and coagulation systems manifest a surgical effect via mechanical oscillation. How is this achieved? Most ultrasonic generators deliver alternating polarity electrical current to an ultrasonic transducer located in the handle of the device that comprises a stack of piezoelectrodes positioned between metal cylinders. When the transducer is activated electrically, the piezoelectrodes are excited and convert the electrical energy to mechanical injury that vibrates the cylinders to create an ultra high-frequency (in the range of 23,000 to 55,500 Hz) linearly oscillating surface that is attached to a solid, contiguous shaft ending in a blade or jaw. Consequently, this blade or jaw oscillates in a linear fashion in concert with the vibrating piezoelectrode.

In most instances, ultrasonic transection or cutting occurs secondary to the mechanical interaction between the oscillating tip of the device and the tissue. In dense tissues, largely comprised of muscle or collagen, or when less dense tissues are compressed or placed on traction, cutting occurs primarily secondary to the mechanical friction created by the oscillating edge of the jaw or blade on the tissue surface. Once the tissue reaches the limit of its elasticity, the blade or jaw is able to create an incision by breaking the protein molecular bonds.

The second method whereby ultrasonic instruments can manifest a cutting effect is via the process of cavitation. For RF electrosurgery and with CO_2 lasers, if sufficient electromagnetic energy is applied the intracellular ions oscillate to the point that the resulting frictional forces cause an elevation of the temperature of the cellular contents to 100°C. At this temperature, the cellular water turns to steam, the intracellular volume increases massively, and the cell ruptures—a process termed vaporization. When the vibrating tip of an ultrasonic surgical instrument is placed in tissue that is less protein- or muscle-dense such as fat, parenchyma or areolar tissue, the intracellular temperatures are raised secondary to the oscillation of the blade, but, in addition, the oscillating tip creates a zone of low atmospheric temperature that effectively reduces the boiling point of the intracellular water. Consequently, cellular vaporization occurs at a much lower temperature than is the case for RF electrosurgery. In these less dense tissues, the gaseous products of cellular vaporization can actually serve to expand the tissue planes, facilitating dissection, a mechanism that, in conjunction with cellular vaporization, gives rise to the term *cavitation*. The cavitation effect enhances visibility in the operative field, which can be especially beneficial in anatomically difficult to reach regions or near vital structures.

Ultrasonically activated instruments can also be used to coagulate tissue, including coaptive coagulation of blood vessels. The ultimate tissue effect is similar to that achieved with the processes of electrosurgical dehydration and protein coagulation, described in Chap. 2. However, the mechanisms whereby cellular and tissue temperature rise are different— with ultrasonic systems, the tissue is heated by external mechanical forces, while with electrosurgery, the temperature elevation occurs secondary to intracellular oscillation of ions, including proteins. So, similar to electrosurgery, coagulation occurs when local temperature increases above 60°C but remains well below 100°C and hydrogen bonds are disrupted, a process that occurs in concert with cellular dehydration.

The disruption in molecular bonds causes denaturation of the protein as the collagen molecules collapse. Along with subsequent cellular and tissue cooling, this results in reformation of the bonds that transforms the tissue into a sticky coagulum. If the surgeon compresses a blood vessel between the jaws of an ultrasonic forceps, for example, the apposed walls of the vessel undergo this process with the result being coaptive coagulation or vessel sealing.

Ultrasonic Surgical Systems

Ultrasonic energy has evolved into a standard operative tool for surgery because of its versatility, effectiveness, and safety. In order to appreciate ultrasonic energy systems, one must be familiar with various components and their purpose.

The Ultrasonic Generator

As described earlier, the ultrasonic generator is used to convert electrical energy into ultrasonic frequency mechanical energy (Figs. 7.1–7.3). The electrical source is typically alternating polarity current from a wall outlet, but some generators rely on constant polarity (direct current) sources such as a lithium battery. The electricity is sent via a cable to an ultrasonic transducer where it is converted by the piezoelectrode into mechanical energy vibrating at a rate of 23–55 kHz.

The amount of mechanical energy applied to tissue per unit time is adjusted by varying the length of excursion of the blade or jaw of the device. Typically, the range of excursion can be adjusted between 50 and 100 μm. Consequently, if the frequency of oscillation is kept constant, a longer blade excursion will transmit more mechanical energy to the adjacent tissue and result in greater cutting efficiency (Figs. 7.1 and 7.2).

Typically, there are two settings available to the surgeon, the maximum excursion (MAX) and a user adjustable excursion (MIN). The MAX setting (larger amount of blade excursion) results in more rapid cutting of tissue and less thermal spread, but also minimizes hemostasis. The "MIN" setting can be adjusted by the surgeon; the reduced excursion of the blade transmits less energy to the tissue per unit time, less efficient cutting, and a greater degree of collateral thermal injury that provides better hemostasis.

LCS - Ligating Cutting Shears

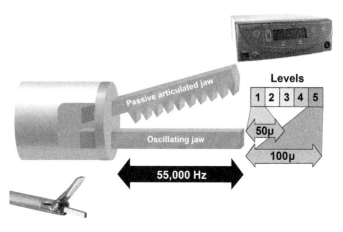

Fig. 7.1. Anatomy of an ultrasonic and sealing device handpiece tip showing the ultrasonic frequency, setting levels (1–5), and active blade excursion.

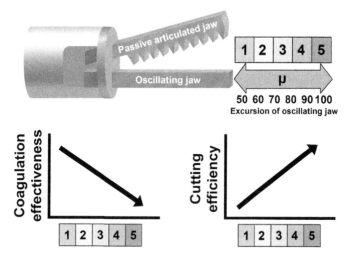

Fig. 7.2. Ultrasonic coagulation and cutting characteristic during blade activation as it relates to power level setting 1 to 5.

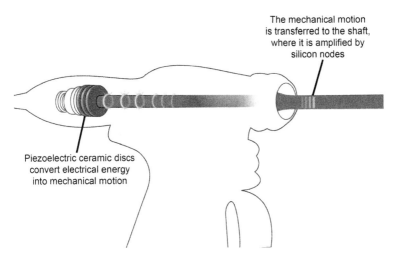

Fig. 7.3. Ultrasonic shears handset contains piezoelectric ceramic discs that convert electrical energy into mechanical motion, which is transferred to the shaft, where it is amplified by silicon nodes.

The Hand Instrument: Ultrasonic Shears

Ultrasonic shears (or ligating cutting devices) comprise a scissor like handle, a shaft that is contiguous with the blade or non-articulated jaw, and an articulated jaw that is controlled by the surgeon by compressing the handle. The handle serves to interface with the ultrasonic generator and the attached piezoelectrode stack. The blade/handle assembly must be firmly attached to the piezoelectrode/cable with mechanisms that vary from system to system.

The articulated jaw opposes the active blade or jaw which can be envisioned as anvil against which the articulated jaw holds and variably compresses the tissue. The greater the pressure, the greater the transmission of frictional and shearing forces; with less pressure there is less cutting and more tissue coagulation (Fig. 7.4).

Clinical Applications of Ultrasonic Shears

Ultrasonic shears can be used to create incisions, perform coaptive coagulation, and transect tissue with minimal lateral thermal spread.

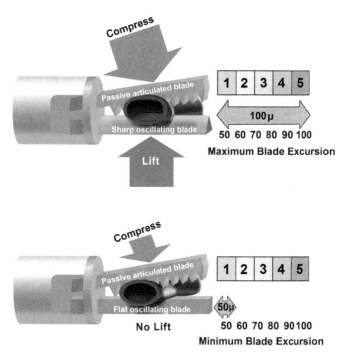

Fig. 7.4. Factors impacting ultrasonic cutting efficiency and coagulation effectiveness during blood vessel coaptation. Compression and lifting provide maximum cutting efficiency and minimum coagulation effectiveness.

However, effective use of the technology requires a set of manual skills that can be easily learned but which are not necessarily intuitive.

Factors that impact the delivery and effect of ultrasonic energy include tissue tension, the power setting (blade excursion) and blade pressure, and jaw sharpness. First of all, ultrasonic shears can be used like a scalpel by opening the jaw allowing the oscillating blade to be applied directly to the tissue. To cut effectively, the tissue must be relatively dense or placed on tension using grasping forceps. More often, the compressive jaw function is employed to provide pressure on the tissue held by the active blade. This pressure adds tension to the tissue that facilitates the mechanical shearing effect increasing the cutting efficiency of the device. Lifting the tissue being cut can create additional tension. The more tension or pressure applied, the more rapid the cutting effect. However with more efficient cutting, there is progressively less tissue coagulation and a greater risk of bleeding if dissecting through vascular tissue. Consequently, the surgeon must operate varying the blade excursion by selecting MIN or MAX and appropriately adjusting the tension on the tissue by varying the pressure of the articulated jaw, and/or the amount of tension applied by lifting the target tissue.

Additional control can be obtained with some ultrasonic shears that have a rotatable blade that can be used to expose the tissue to a sharp edge, a rounded edge, or a flat edge. In this way, the hemostatic tissue effect can be enhanced or reduced by blade configuration in a manner analogous to the active electrode tip designs for electrosurgery (i.e., the broader the blade, the more coagulation effect).

Ultrasonic energy devices are used in open and laparoscopic operations, and come in various lengths, diameters, and configurations. Frequent instrument tip configurations include straight, curved, and hook blades. Shaft lengths range from 16 cm to 45 cm, the later length necessary for patients with clinically severe obesity. Maximum blade temperature can reach 105°C with widest thermal spread of approximately 3 mm according to published studies. Data from multiple, independent, *in vivo* and *ex vivo* animal studies in which vessel sealing devices were tested on arteries of various diameters according to manufacturer specifications demonstrated that arterial burst pressure and burst failure rate vary by vessel and device diameters tested, generators used, and study methodology employed. Average arterial burst pressures ranged from 204 mmHg to 1,071 mmHg while average burst failure rates were 8% to 39%.

Advantages and Disadvantages of Ultrasonic Shears

It is imperative that surgeons and allied health professionals understand not only the advantages but also the disadvantages of ultrasonic energy devices. The advantages of ultrasonic devices are multiple and include hemostasis and division of unsupported vascular tissues ≤5 mm in diameter. Ultrasonic shears also offer versatility as a tool that grasps, dissects, cuts, and coagulates tissue. This versatility may result in fewer instrument exchanges during procedures, particularly in laparoscopic surgery. By using the active blade alone, one can mimic the effect of a monopolar electrosurgical electrode. No tissue sticking occurs because of the vibrations of the active blade on the tissue and the lower heat generated at the blade–tissue interface. Minimal thermal injury occurs as a function of the energy type and mechanics of the ultrasonic shears, a feature that makes the ultrasonic shears well-suited for the creation of enterotomies, gastrostomies, or colotomies prior to anastomosis.

There is no need to apply a dispersive electrode, and, more importantly, the absence of an electrical current passing through the patient's body eliminates complications of monopolar electrosurgical instrumentation such as alternate site burns and current diversion from insulation defects, or direct or capacitive coupling.

There are a number of disadvantages of ultrasonic shears that must be considered when contemplating their use. As previously described, vascular sealing is dependent upon accurate application of the energy, which can be very surgeon dependent. As with electrosurgical devices, tissue sticking can occur when eschar accumulates on the jaws necessitating cleaning the blades by activating the device in saline or water. Blade fatigue or fracture can occur with prolonged or inappropriate use of the device and may be suspected with poor functionality or by system alarms.

Perhaps the most important risk associated with the use of ultrasonic surgical cutting and coagulating devices, including ultrasonic shears, is related to the heat that can be retained in the shaft, particularly after prolonged activation. Depending on the target tissue, the shaft or blade of the device may retain a "kill" temperature ($\geq 60°C$) for about 20 s when activating in liver and up to 45 s when the target tissue is mesentery or peritoneum. Indeed, the duration of retention of this temperature is very prolonged compared to bipolar electrosurgical instruments. Consequently, if for example, the ureter or small bowel comes in contact with the active blade of the ultrasonic device during activation or immediately following activation and before an adequate cooling period, a full-thickness injury can occur. Safety methods to prevent injury from the extreme temperature of the active blade include careful activation of the device under direct visualization and refraining from manipulation and dissection of tissues without allowing for a cooling period. General differences between electrosurgical devices and ultrasonic shears are listed in Table 7.1.

Summary

While ultrasonic energy systems are increasingly employed as a means to dissect, cut, and coagulate tissues and a growing body of research across disciplines supports the efficacy of ultrasonic energy, the

Table 7.1. Differences between electrosurgery devices and ultrasonic shears.

Category	Electrosurgery	Ultrasonic shears
Grounding electrode	Yes	No
Smoke generation	Yes	No
Electrocardiogram, pacemaker interference	Yes	No
Current travels through patient	Yes	No
Heat generation	Constant	Time dependent
Thermal spread	Moderate	Minimal
Cost	Low/Intermediate	Intermediate/High
Complications	Current concentration Direct coupling Capacitive coupling Tissue sticking	Thermal injury

value of these devices depends on their safe use. This chapter addresses the basic principles of mechanical energy and the fundamentals for the use of safe ultrasonic energy by describing the components of ultrasonic energy systems, the potential complications of ultrasonic energy use, and methods to prevent or reduce injury.

References

1. Bandi G, Wen CC, Wilkinson EA, Hedican SP, Moon TD, Nakada SY. Comparison of blade temperature dynamics after activation of Harmonic ACE scalpel and the Ultracision Harmonic Scalpel LCS-K5. J Endourol. 2008;22:333–6.
2. Campbell PA, Cresswell AB, Frank TG, Cuschieri FA. Real-time thermography during energized vessel sealing and dissection. Surg Endosc. 2003;17:1640–5.
3. Clements RH, Paiepu R. In vivo comparison of the coagulation capability of SonoSurg and Harmonic Ace on 4 mm and 5 mm arteries. Surg Endosc. 2007;21:2203–6.
4. Gandsas A, Adrales GL. Energy sources. In: Talamini MA, editor. Advanced therapy in minimally invasive surgery. Lewiston, NY: BC Decker; 2006. p. 3–9.
5. Hruby GW, Marruffo FC, Durak E, et al. Evaluation of surgical energy devices for vessel sealing and peripheral energy spread in a porcine model. J Urol. 2007;178: 2689–93.
6. Kim FJ, Chammas Jr MF, Gewehr E, et al. Temperature safety profile of laparoscopic devices: Harmonic ACE (ACE), Ligasure V (LV), and plasma trisector (PT). Surg Endosc. 2008;22:1464–9.
7. Lamberton GR, His RS, Jin DH, Lindler TU, Jellison FC, Baldwin DD. Prospective comparison of four laparoscopic vessel ligation devices. J Endourol. 2008;22: 2307–12.

8. Newcomb WL, Hope WW, Schmelzer TM, et al. Comparison of blood vessel sealing among new electrosurgical and ultrasonic devices. Surg Endosc. 2009;23:90–6.

9. Newman RM, Traverso LW. Principles of laparoscopic hemostasis. In: Scott-Conner CEH, editor. The SAGES manual: fundamentals of laparoscopy, thoracoscopy, and GI endoscopy. 2nd ed. New York, NY: Springer; 2006. p. 49–59.

10. Person B, Vivas DA, Ruiz D, Talcott M, Coad JE, Wexner SD. Comparison of four energy-based vascular sealing and cutting instruments: a porcine model. Surg Endosc. 2008;22:534–8.

11. Phillips CK, Hruby GW, Durak E, et al. Tissue response to surgical energy devices. Urology. 2008;71:744–8.

8. Cavitron Ultrasonic Surgical Aspirator

James S. Choi

Different techniques of liver parenchymal transection have been described, including finger fracture, sharp dissection, clamp-crush technique, the hydrojet, and more recently, the Cavitron Ultrasonic Surgical Aspirator (CUSA). The CUSA is an innovative tool for dissecting through the liver parenchyma, which can potentially reduce intraoperative blood loss and perioperative morbidity. The CUSA system is a powerful ultrasonic aspirator and dissector with application in liver surgery and other surgical specialties as well. The CUSA system consists of a handpiece and a main control unit (console) to which the handpiece is connected.

The CUSA is used in multiple surgical subspecialties, including neurosurgery, gastrointestinal, hepatobiliary surgery, gynecology, and urology. CUSA Excel is an ultrasonic surgical aspirator enabling fragmentation, suction, and irrigation to occur simultaneously, allowing the surgeon to remove tissue with accurate control. In liver surgery, it can be an invaluable tool, particularly in a situation where the tumor is closely adjacent to a vital structure that needs to be saved. CUSA will enable dissection around structures that needs to be preserved.

Tissue Fragmentation

The CUSA device allows the user to fragment organ tissues. When fragmenting parenchymal tissue, it leaves structures such as blood vessels and ducts intact. Tissue strength affects both the fragmentation rate and the ability of any ultrasonic aspirator handpiece to remove tissue. Tissues

L.S. Feldman et al. (eds.), *The SAGES Manual on the Fundamental
Use of Surgical Energy (FUSE)*, DOI 10.1007/978-1-4614-2074-3_8,
© Springer Science+Business Media, LLC 2012

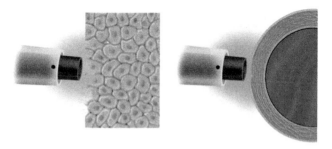

Fig. 8.1. CUSA effect on low-strength tissue (*left*) and high-strength tissue (*right*). The differential effect is due to the different amount of high-strength intercellular bonds in tissue, and is exploited in the CUSA technique to dissect liver parenchyma without injuring vessels and bile ducts.

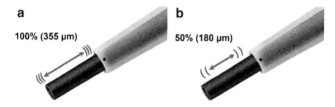

Fig. 8.2. (**a**) High amplitude. (**b**) Low amplitude. The tissue effect of CUSA can be modulated, as the speed of fragmentation depends on the amplitude setting, which determines the distance of tip stroke.

with weak intracellular bonds (low-strength) are the easiest to fragment, and include tissues with moderate or high fluid content, such as some tumors, parenchyma, and fat. Tissues with strong intracellular bonds (high-strength) are the most difficult to fragment, and include vessel walls, ducts, nerves, tendons, ligaments, and organ capsules. These structures contain less fluid and more collagen and/or elastin, which provide resistance to fragmentation (Fig. 8.1).

The speed of fragmentation depends on the amplitude setting, which determines the distance of the tip stroke. The higher the amplitude, the longer the tip stroke—resulting in a greater impact force that produces a higher fragmentation rate. Conversely, the lower amplitude produces a shorter stroke, less impact force, and a slower fragmentation rate (Fig. 8.2).

Mechanics

The CUSA console provides alternating current (23 or 36 kHz) to the handpiece. In the handpiece, the current passes through a coil, which induces a magnetic field. The magnetic field in turn excites a transducer of nickel alloy laminations, resulting in oscillating motion in the transducer laminated structure—vibration—along its long axis. The transducer transmits vibrations through a metal connecting body to an attached surgical tip. When the vibrating tip contacts tissue, it breaks cells apart (fragmentation). The CUSA system supports both 23 and 36 kHz magnetostrictive handpieces, and each supports multiple tip designs. The powerful 23 kHz handpiece fragments even tough, fibrous, and calcified tumors while the small, 36 kHz handpiece is helpful during procedures requiring precision, tactile feedback, and delicate control. A wide variety of tips enables customization of the handpiece for each procedure, depending on the consistency, location, and depth of the targeted tissue.

Irrigation and Suction

The CUSA has a self-contained suction capability to remove fragmented tissue and irrigation fluid. Suction power is generated directly from the CUSA unit, and it ensures that the suction power is consistent and the maximum possible. Consistent, strong suction provides two major benefits in ultrasonic aspiration. First, it draws tissue toward the vibrating tip, and creates a tip/tissue coupling effect. Second, it keeps the surgical site clear of irrigation and fragmentation debris and minimizes blockage in the suction tubing. Irrigation fluid flows coaxillary around the outside of the vibrating tip to keep the tip cool and to suspend fragmented tissue in solution to minimize tip blockage (Fig. 8.3).

A clear, silicone flue encircles the tip and provides a continuous pathway for delivery of the irrigation fluid. The flue ends approximately 2 mm from the distal end of the tip and just covers the pre-aspiration holes. The two 0.4-mm holes aspirate as much as 95% of the irrigation fluid back through the inside of the hollow tip before the fluid reaches the end of the tip and the surgical site. The pre-aspiration holes have several functions: (1) Removing the heat generated by the rapidly vibrating tip to help prevent tip fracture and thermal tissue damage. (2) Lubricating and suspending

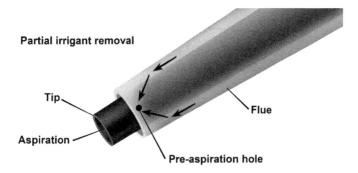

Fig. 8.3. Detailed description of the active CUSA tip. For details see text.

the fragmented tissue to prevent blockage in the suction line. (3) Reducing the amount of irrigant delivered to the surgical site to eliminate the flooding and fluid bubbling that may interfere with visibility.

Cooling

The high-frequency vibration generates heat. To reduce the heat, the CUSA system includes a closed, recirculating cooling water circuit. The pump circulates water from a reservoir to and through the tube in the handpiece, then to the return tube in the handpiece and back to the reservoir. As the water moves through the handpiece, it removes heat. The CUSA suction pathway is completely external, so fragmented tissue and fluids never flow through the inside of the handpiece. The tip and suction tubing that come into contact with fragmented tissue are disposable.

Pitfalls

When handling the CUSA, it is very important to remember a few basic points about the dangers of the device. First, it is important to remember how to hold the handpiece. It is best held like a pen/pencil. It is very important to remember not to squeeze the flue which can restrict the flow of irrigation fluid, which in turn will result in frictional heating and potential burning of the surgeon's hand (Fig. 8.4). When performing

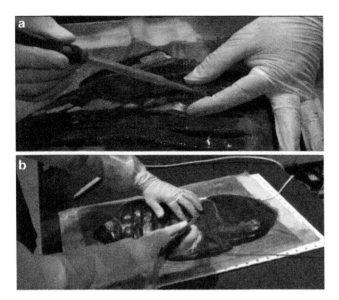

Fig. 8.4. (**a, b**) Correct hand and instrument position of the CUSA for dissection of liver tissue. *Upper panel* shows correct hold of instrument and *lower panel* application to liver parenchyma. See text for details.

liver resections with the CUSA device, it is very important to remember that while vessel walls are relatively difficult to fragment, much of the veins in the liver are very thin and fragile, so any manipulation may potentially result in catastrophic bleeding. It is therefore good practice to use the CUSA in such a way as to not fragment too much tissue too quickly. Particular care should be taken when dissecting around major blood vessels.

References

1. Chan KK, Watmough DJ, Hope DT, Moir K. A new motor-driven surgical probe and its in vitro comparison with the Cavitron Ultrasonic Surgical Aspirator. Ultrasound Med Biol. 1986;12(4):279–83.
2. Chopp RT, Shah BB, Addonizio JC. Use of ultrasonic surgical aspirator in renal surgery. Urology. 1983;22(2):157–9.
3. Deppe G, Malviya VK, Malone Jr JM. Use of Cavitron Ultrasonic Surgical Aspirator (CUSA) for palliative resection of recurrent gynecologic malignancies involving the vagina. Eur J Gynaecol Oncol. 1989;10(1):1–2.

4. Deppe G, Malviya VK, Malone Jr JM. Debulking surgery for ovarian cancer with the Cavitron Ultrasonic Surgical Aspirator (CUSA)—a preliminary report. Gynecol Oncol. 1988;31(1):223–6.
5. Farid H, O'Connell T. Hepatic resections: changing mortality and morbidity. Am Surg. 1994;60(10):748–52.
6. Fasulo F, Giori A, Fissi S, Bozzetti F, Doci R, Gennari L. Cavitron Ultrasonic Surgical Aspirator (CUSA) in liver resection. Int Surg. 1992;77(1):64–6.
7. Freysdottir D, Nielsson J, Magnusson J. Hepatic resections. The results of using CUSA. Laeknabladid. 1994;80(9):465–70.
8. Hardy KJ, Martin J, Fletcher DR, MacLellan DG, Jones RM. Hepatic resection: value of operative ultrasound and ultrasonic dissection. Aust N Z J Surg. 1989;59(8):621–3.
9. Koo BN, Kil HK, Choi JS, Kim JY, Chun DH, Hong YW. Hepatic resection by the Cavitron Ultrasonic Surgical Aspirator increases the incidence and severity of venous air embolism. Anesth Analg. 2005;101(4):966–70.
10. Lee JH, Kwon TD, Kim HJ, Kang B, Koo BN. Multiple cerebral infarction and paradoxical air embolism during hepatectomy using the Cavitron Ultrasonic Surgical Aspirator—a case report. Korean J Anesthesiol. 2010;59(Suppl):S133–6.
11. Little JM, Hollands MJ. Impact of the CUSA and operative ultrasound on hepatic resection. HPB Surg. 1991;3(4):271–7.
12. Morishita Y, Konishi I, Noda Y, Mori T. Usage of the CUSA (cavitron ultrasonic surgical aspirator) in radical surgery of cervical carcinoma of the uterus. Gan To Kagaku Ryoho. 1987;14(5):1494–500.
13. Nagano Y, Matsuo K, Kunisaki C, Ike H, Imada T, Tanaka K, Togo S, Shimada H. Practical usefulness of ultrasonic surgical aspirator with argon beam coagulation for hepatic parenchymal transaction. World J Surg. 2005;29(7):899–902.
14. Pamecha V, Gurusamy KS, Sharma D, Davidson BR. Techniques for liver parenchymal transaction: a meta-analysis of randomized controlled trials. HPB. 2009;11(4):275–81.
15. Storck BH, Rutgers EJ, Gortzak E, Zoetmulder FA. The impact of the CUSA ultrasonic dissection device on major liver resections. Neth J Surg. 1991;43(4):99–101.
16. Yamamoto Y, Ikai L, Kume M, Sakai Y, et al. New simple technique for hepatic parenchymal resection using a Cavitron Ultrasonic Surgical Aspirator and bipolar cautery equipped with a channel for water dripping. World J Surg. 1999;23(10):1032–7.

9. Principles and Safety of Radiofrequency and Cryo Ablation

Pascal R. Fuchshuber

Radiofrequency ablation (RFA) is a subset (special form) of radiofrequency electrosurgery (see Chap. 2) developed to coagulate and thereby destroy large volumes of tissue. The word *ablation* is misleading as it stands for a technique of "layer by layer removal" of tissue. A better description of ablation in the context of RFA is thermal coagulation of a large volume of tissue. However, the terminology *RFA* is well established and is used in this chapter to describe large volume thermal ablation of tissue with radiofrequency current. To be optimally effective at ablating such large tissue volumes, RF Ablation systems are designed to achieve local cellular and tissue temperatures that result only in electrosurgical coagulation while avoiding temperatures that result in tissue vaporization and carbonization, the latter a consequence of local temperatures greater than 200°C.

RFA coexists with other nonresectional techniques based on non-RF technologies such as microwave (see Chap. 10), tissue freezing, or focused ultrasound. The focus of this chapter is on the basic principles and techniques of RFA and its safety as it pertains to its clinical application. It does not cover the different proprietary types of RFA systems currently available nor does it discuss all clinical applications, treatment algorithms, and outcomes.

Basic Principles

RFA is based on the application of alternating current at a frequency of 375–500 kHz (radiofrequency) through an active electrode placed into the target tissue (Fig. 9.1). The process is based on the principles described in Chap. 2. To summarize, the alternating polarity of the output from the electrosurgical unit (ESU) results in rapid oscillation

L.S. Feldman et al. (eds.), *The SAGES Manual on the Fundamental Use of Surgical Energy (FUSE)*, DOI 10.1007/978-1-4614-2074-3_9, © Springer Science+Business Media, LLC 2012

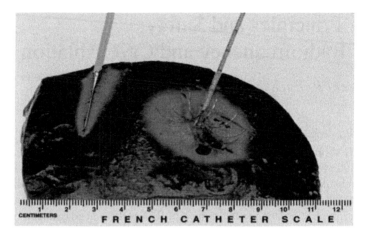

Fig. 9.1. Volumetric RF ablation: A single electrode provides a limited amount of tissue destruction (*left*) compared to the multitined RF Ablation instrument that combines multiple electrodes simultaneously creating a much larger zone of tissue coagulation and desiccation (*right*).

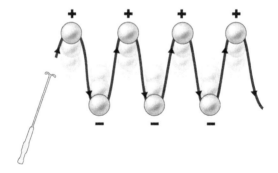

Fig. 9.2. Alternating current at a frequency of 375–500 kHz is applied through an active electrode. The oscillating current creates an alternating electric field that leads to ionic agitation and subsequent frictional heat. The generated heat leads to destruction of the target tissue.

of intracellular ions, including proteins (Fig. 9.2). This oscillation occurs at a rate that is synchronous with the frequency of the ESU output and the resulting frictional forces quickly increase the intracellular temperature in the tissue surrounding the active electrode(s). If this temperature reaches 60°C—and if it remains below 100°C—the simultaneous processes of protein coagulation and tissue desiccation occur, leading to cellular death and tissue destruction. In principle RFA systems are designed to produce a specific power output through proprietary algorithms that allow for thermal coagulation of a maximum tissue volume by preventing premature tissue desiccation. This is done by downregulating power output to maximize heating of tissue *before* desiccation resulting in rapid increase of impedance (resistance) occurs. This rapid increase in impedance will limit the volume of thermal coagulation and lead to a less than desired amount of tissue destruction.

The relatively high power (or current) concentration around the active electrode is related to its relatively small surface area. The other electrode in the system, the dispersive electrode, distributes the same current over a much larger area—with a much lower power density. As a result, no tissue effect should occur at the dispersive electrode. However, some RF ablation systems produce so much power that the current density in a single dispersive electrode can reach a level that would result in thermal injury to the underlying skin. The solution to this problem is to reduce the power density further with the application of several dispersive electrodes. In such cases, additional safety is provided by continuously measuring the local temperature at the dispersive electrode to ensure that temperature levels associated with skin injury are not achieved [1, 2].

Monopolar RFA systems use a design in which the patient is part of a closed-loop circuit with an electrosurgical generator or unit (ESU), an active electrode or an array of active electrodes, and one or more large dispersive electrodes (Fig. 9.3). Each of the active electrodes has a small surface area compared to that of the large dispersive electrodes. This focuses the RF current on the interface between the active electrode(s) and the target tissue, while at the dispersive electrode—tissue interface the same current is diffused so that no or only moderate temperature elevation occurs. The entire patient is interposed between the active and the dispersive electrodes. In bipolar RFA system, the instrument contains both of the required electrodes, each of which is "active," and, because they are placed in close proximity to each other, both contribute to the thermal effect within the target tissue. In general monopolar designs lead to wider ablation zones around the active electrode and are easier to manipulate as there is only one instrument (active electrode) to be placed. Bipolar designs achieve better focusing of the energy between the two active electrodes and obviate the need for a dispersive electrode and its associated possible complications. There are several monopolar and one bipolar RFA system currently available for clinical use. This chapter is limited to the description of monopolar systems as the basic principles are similar for both systems, and most currently available ESUs for RF ablation are designed to work with monopolar instruments.

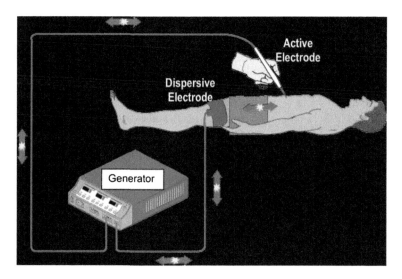

Fig. 9.3. Monopolar RFA system: the patient is part of a closed-loop circuit with a generator, an active electrode and one or more large dispersive electrodes.

Thermal destruction of the target tissue by RFA occurs at 50°C or higher (see Chap. 2). At 50°C the time to irreversible cellular damage is approximately 6 min. At 60°C or higher cellular death is instantaneous. Above 60°C protein denaturation as well as dehydration or desiccation occurs. At 100°C water boils and tissue vaporizes with production of steam. At temperatures over 200°C tissues carbonize. These effects dictate the optimal temperature range of 50–100°C for RFA as below 50°C cell death does not occur and above 100°C steam formation disrupts the contact between the tissues and the active electrode thus impeding the desired effect on the target tissue. Similarly, charring around the active electrode at temperatures above 200°C counteracts the ablation process. Intracellular heating of the target tissue by RF current occurs only within a few millimeters of the active electrode. The majority of the final ablation zone is created due to thermal conduction away from the active electrode. Heat from the ablation zone immediately adjacent to the tines of the active electrode(s) is distributed deeper into the target tissue by heat conduction. This process takes time and it is critical that deposition of energy immediately around the active electrode resulting from ion agitation due to conduction of RF current continues during this time. Therefore, it is critical that tissue desiccation, vaporization, and carbonization do *not* occur early in the process of RF ablation as this would create an "insulator" around the active electrode(s) and impede the conductive propagation of heat throughout the target tissue. An incomplete ablation would be the result. Several effects determine the success of an RF ablation in this context:

1. For ionic agitation to occur tissue must contain ions in a fluid state. Thus the water content of the target is critical to the ability to generate heat and subsequent cellular destruction. Low water content or desiccation increases resistance to electrical current and reduces heat production. Thus RFA is a self-limiting process as desiccation eventually occurs.

2. High tissue resistance or impedance due to formation of steam or charring will stop the ablation process. Therefore, the goal of RFA is to keep the temperature around the active electrode below 100°C for as long as possible to allow deposition of heat for as long as possible in order to obtain the largest possible ablation zone. An analogy to trying to cook a well-done hamburger patty comes to mind: rapid heating causes carbonization of the outside surface and prevents the raw center to cook.

In physical terms, the RFA system needs to adjust the delivery of energy to the impedance present at the active electrode/target tissue interface to prevent too rapid heating and to prolong deposition of thermal energy for as long as possible. This is achieved by constant measurement of the impedance and/or temperature and by adjusting the delivered electrical power (wattage) to achieve the lowest possible impedance at a tissue temperature of 50–100°C (Fig. 9.4). There are several proprietary

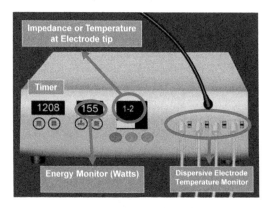

Fig. 9.4. Basic design of ESU for RFA. Energy and impedance or temperature at the active electrode is constantly monitored and adjusted to provide maximum delivery of heat without causing early desiccation or carbonization.

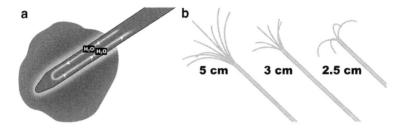

Fig. 9.5. Different proprietary designs of electrodes with the same goal in mind: maximizing deposition of energy over time while minimizing charring or vaporization. Shown are electrode designs that use cooling (**a**) and multiple tines (**b**) to prevent excessive heat production and thus charring immediately around the active electrode.

RFA systems on the market that achieve this with different algorithms and active electrode designs (Fig. 9.5). In most systems the voltage is kept constant and at a low threshold of around 60 V. This voltage threshold is below the voltage that can induce sparks and thus charring. In order to ablate large amounts of tissue, the delivered electrical energy can reach 250 W. This energy level requires large dispersive electrodes and newer systems can have multiple dispersive electrodes to prevent skin burns due to high energy density.

General Technique

To ensure a successful ablation, the active electrode is optimally placed into the target lesion under image guidance, by using either ultrasound or CT/MRI assistance. It is critical to be well-versed in image-guided techniques when using an RFA system, i.e., a surgeon should be trained in intraoperative US. The optimal placement of the active electrode depends on the design of each proprietary system. It is important to know the specific results expected with each proprietary design and follow the instruction for optimal electrode placement into the target [3]. Once the active electrode is connected to a radiofrequency generator and activated, the target lesion is heated using a proprietary device-specific algorithm until a specific target is reached. This target can be either the rise of tissue impedance (resistance to the electrical current) or a target tissue temperature measured by the electrode in situ.

The obvious goal of RFA is complete destruction of the target tissue. The size of the ablation zone and thus the complete destruction of the target tissue are determined by the properties of the target tissue and the surrounding tissue. The effect of RFA is determined by the electrical and thermal conductivity of the tissues. Electrical conductivity is inversely proportional to the resistance or impedance of the tissue. High water content reduces resistance and increases conductivity. High water content also increases thermal diffusion through the tissue. As an example the determining factors that apply to RF ablations in livers are discussed here:

1. *The time during which ionic agitation and thermal conduction occur.* Since a substantial portion of RF ablation requires heat conduction through the target tissue away from the zone of direct RF energy-induced ionic agitation immediately around the active electrode, total ablation time needs to be sufficient to allow this process to be effective and heat all target tissue. It is important to follow the proprietary algorithm of each system in this respect.

2. *The even deposition of energy* (Figs. 9.6 and 9.7). The direct electromagnetic effect of RFA occurs only within a few millimeters of the active electrode. The majority of the energy is deposited by thermal diffusion and dependent on the thermal conductivity of the target tissue. Propagation of heat from the active electrode is uneven due to small difference in

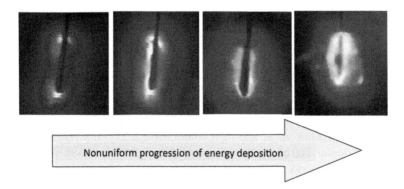

Fig. 9.6. Slow irregular progression of energy deposition in the form of heat immediately adjacent to an active electrode during RFA. (Copyright 2010 Covidien. All rights reserved. Reprinted with the permission of the Energy Based Division of Covidien).

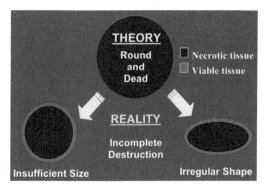

Fig. 9.7. In most clinical situations, an even spherical RF ablation remains theoretical. In practice, the shape of ablation zones is irregular with the threat of insufficient size and thus incomplete ablation.

the electrical and thermal conductive properties of the target lesion and the surrounding tissue. It is critical to be mindful of this and allow ample time for complete ablation of the target lesion.

3. *The size and shape of the target lesion.* Most target lesions do not have an ideal spherical shape and one should take into account the typical ablation zone created by a particular proprietary design of an active electrode. Multiple ablations of a single odd-shaped target lesion might be necessary to assure complete destruction.

4. *The tissue properties of the target lesion.* Because RF ablation relies on ionic agitation within the target tissue, high water content facilitates this process as more ions are in solution and can participate in the generation of heat. High water content improves ablation results as a higher amount of RF energy can be deposited into the tissue before they desiccate. Desiccation increases impedance (lowers electrical conductivity) and decreases thermal diffusion. For example, a target lesion with low water and high connective tissue content such as a colorectal cancer metastasis will be more difficult to ablate with RF energy while a neuroendocrine metastasis with high water content is easier to ablate.

5. *The tissue properties of the surrounding tissue.* The water content and therefore the perfusion-mediated cooling effect of the tissue surrounding the target lesion directly impact the

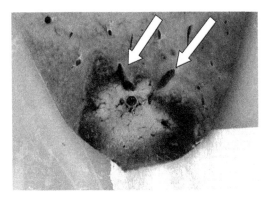

Fig. 9.8. Large vessels (hepatic veins, *white arrows*) cause irregular ablation zone and can compromise the intended destruction of the target lesion.

effectiveness of the RF Ablation. Low water content or low perfusion of the surrounding tissue will aid the ablation process and prevent thermal diffusion away from the target lesion. For example, ablation of a target lesion in a cirrhotic liver will be more efficient and completed in a shorter time than in a normal liver. Application of the Pringle maneuver (vascular clamping of the inflow of blood into the liver) decreases the thermal conductivity of the surrounding tissue and has been shown to increase the size of the ablation zone in experimental models and is commonly used when large ablations are desired in hepatic target lesions [4].

6. *The presence of large blood vessels adjacent to the target lesion* (Figs. 9.8 and 9.9). Large blood vessels in the immediate vicinity to a target lesion may cause an electrical sink due to diversion of current through the path of least resistance or by heat sink through faster and more efficient convection of heat through an adjacent blood vessel. Knowledge of the particular anatomy at the ablation site is therefore of critical importance.

RF ablations are performed in many different organs such as bone, kidney, and lung. Each of these organs may require special considerations for optimal ablations. Ablations can be performed percutaneously, laparoscopically, or with open surgical exposure and each of these techniques requires special skills and particular imaging modalities. Those aspects of RF ablation techniques are not subject of this chapter.

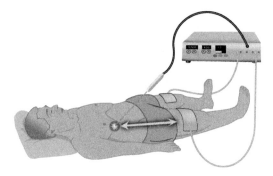

Fig. 9.9. Correct placement of dispersive electrodes when using a monopolar RFA system. The long axis of the dispersive electrode is at a right angle to the direction of the current flow and away from the heart. Presence of metal implants need to be taken into account. Some systems use more than one dispersive electrode to accommodate current density and avoid thermal injury.

Safety

RFA is a complex procedure using high energy monopolar or bipolar systems delivering up to 250 W. Safety issues can be divided in those related to injuries to operator and patient and those related to the inappropriate technical application. The other aspect of safety is related to its clinical goal of complete destruction of the target lesion. Clinical safety in this context is principally oncological safety and prevention of tumor recurrence.

Operator and Patient Safety

For the prevention of injury and maximum safety, it is important that someone in the operating room besides the surgeon understands the device and knows how to use it correctly. The adequacy of function of the RFA system should be part of the preoperative checklist. Next the adequate number and placement of dispersive electrodes must be ascertained. Up to four dispersive electrodes are used with certain systems to assure adequate dispersion of the large amount of energy used. Even within one proprietary system different dispersive electrodes are prescribed depending on what type of active electrode is used. The availability of the appropriate active and dispersive electrode needs to be assessed prior to the start of the operation. The connections of the active and dispersive electrodes to the generator also need to be checked for functionality so that the feedback mechanisms through the active electrode for measuring adequacy of ablation and the temperature monitoring of the dispersive electrode are functional.

Because a large amount of energy is used in RFA, dispersive electrodes can heat up significantly and cause thermal injury to the patient. It is imperative that the dispersive electrodes are placed correctly on the patient. Orientation and position with regard to the site of ablation and anatomic consideration are crucial. The dispersive electrode should be placed away from the heart or metal implants. The orientation of the electrode needs to take into account the direction of current flow and the long axis of the electrode is placed in a right angle to the current flow (Fig. 9.9). Any contact with the dispersive electrode needs to be avoided during the operation as distortion of the electrode configuration, for example by leaning with one's elbow on it, can cause a "hotspot" at the skin interface and severe skin burns. For this reason some proprietary systems have build-in temperature monitoring systems for the dispersive electrodes.

Additional unintended injuries can occur due to the heat generated at the ablation site (Table 9.1). The patient can experience mild hyperthermia with prolonged ablation and is not life threatening. Because of the heat generated, injury to structures adjacent to the target lesion and to organs adjacent to the target organ may occur. For example, in liver ablation potentially life-threatening injuries to biliary and vascular structures and

Table 9.1. Most common complications of RFA.

Injury	How to prevent	Potentially life threatening
Hyperthermia	Monitor intraoperative core temperature	No
Skin burns	Correct placement of dispersive electrode	No
Vascular injury	Avoid excessive ablation close to large vessels	Yes
Biliary injury	Avoid ablation close to liver hilum	Yes
Organ injury	Create space between liver surface and adjacent organ	Yes
Diaphragmatic injury	Create space between liver surface and diaphragm	Yes
Liver abscess	Do not ablate with biliary obstruction or cholangitis	Yes
Tumor rupture/seeding	Avoid ablation of large surface lesions	No

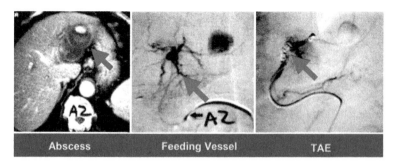

Fig. 9.10. Postablation hematoma with abscess. Angiogram shows feeding vessel and subsequent successful trans-arterial-embolization is shown on the right. (Courtesy of Dr. Anton Bilchik).

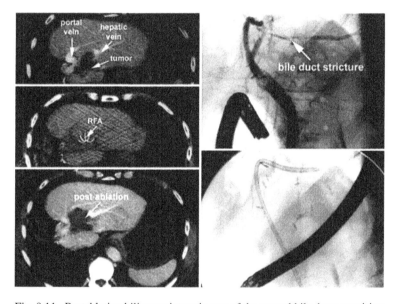

Fig. 9.11. Postablation biliary stricture in one of the central bile ducts requiring ERCP-stent placement. Picture on the *left* shows the ablation sequence, pictures on the *right* the biliary stricture and subsequent stent placement. (Courtesy of Dr. Anton Bilchik).

to organs adjacent to the liver can occur. In general these injuries are too small to be recognized or cause problems. Serious injuries are described with vascular injuries that cause large hematomas requiring embolization (Fig. 9.10) and biliary injuries requiring internal or external stenting (Fig. 9.11). Injuries to adjacent organs during ablation of surface lesions of the liver for example can cause heat-induced necrosis and can be initially difficult to diagnose. Because of the risk of perforation of intestine or stomach, these injuries can on rare occasions result in sepsis and even death. Diaphragmatic injuries may require operative repair. Abscess formation within the necrotic ablation zone is not uncommon and may require drainage.

The overall rate of these complications of RFA is less than 5% and depends on the type of approach used: in general complications are higher with percutaneous techniques due to the inability to separate adjacent organs from the target organ such as the liver. Targeting with percutaneous techniques may also be less accurate than with laparoscopic or open surgical techniques [5, 6].

Prevention of these injuries can be achieved most often through careful attention to the target lesion's location in relationship to vital structures such as bile ducts and to adjacent organs. This requires excellent imaging modalities during ablation procedures such as intraoperative ultrasound or CT/MRI guidance.

Oncologic Safety

Oncologic safety essentially is the avoidance of tumor recurrence after RFA. Local recurrence after ablation is due to incomplete destruction of the target tissue (Fig. 9.12). As previously discussed, the RFA process is uneven due to the properties of the target tissue and the surrounding tissue. In general, the larger the target lesion and the closer its association to large vessels the more likely an incomplete ablation will occur (Fig. 9.13). The type of technique used (percutaneous vs. surgical) can influence recurrence rates as well [7]. It is critical to follow the proprietary algorithm for each system and to ensure correct ablation time. As a rule, the targeted ablation zone should exceed the size of the target lesion by at least 1 cm circumferentially (Fig. 9.14). Adequate assessment of the size and shape of the target lesion prior ablation and correct placement of the active electrode is essential.

Because of the significant risk of incomplete ablation with reported rates of up to 28% for liver tumors [8], the indications for RFA have been relatively narrow:

1. Palliative intent for pain or bridge to transplant.
2. Surgically unresectable lesions because of location or overall tumor burden [9].
3. Poor surgical candidate.

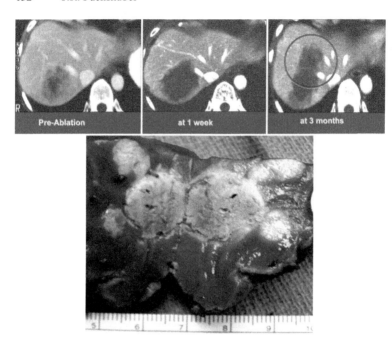

Fig. 9.12. Local recurrence after RFA of liver tumors. *Top* shows evolution of ablation zone over time with development of a local recurrence (*red circle*). *Bottom* shows excision specimen after tumor recurrence in the periphery of an ablated liver lesion.

Cryoablation

Cryoablation describes a process by which tissue is destroyed through freezing. This is achieved by circulating very cold fluids (liquid nitrogen) through hollow needles (cryoprobes) that have been placed into the target tissue to be destroyed. Cryoablation, in contrast to RFA, achieves tissue destruction by freezing tissue. Tissue death occurs through the disruption of cellular membranes by ice crystals within the cellular and extracellular matrix. Additional mechanisms that lead to tissue destruction are coagulation of blood in small capillaries and induction of apoptosis by very low temperatures.

Similar to RFA, the active probes (cryoprobes) are placed through various imaging techniques (ultrasound, CT, MRI) into the target tissue. In contrast to RFA the progress of the cryoablation can be monitored in real time with ultrasound. Cryoablation is most commonly used to destroy

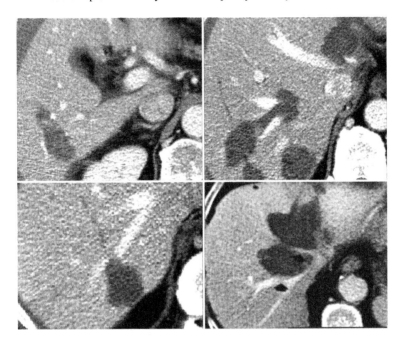

Fig. 9.13. Irregular ablation zones due to ablation close to vessels, increasing the risk of an incomplete ablation during RFA. (Courtesy of Dr. S. Curley).

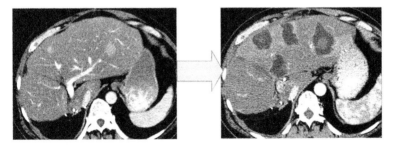

Fig. 9.14. Demonstration of two cases with adequate ablation zones. Shown is at least a 1 cm circumferential overlap of the target lesion after RFA of malignant liver lesions (*left* before RFA, *right* after RFA).

solid tumors of the lung, liver, breast, kidney, and prostate. It can be applied with both laparoscopic and open surgical techniques. However, today it is most commonly performed percutaneously by interventional radiologists or by cardiologists for ablation of abnormal pacing tissue in the heart.

The feared complications of uncontrolled hemorrhage because of disseminated coagulopathy were seen with first generation large bore cryoprobes in open surgical procedures, particularly in the liver. These life-threatening complications are not seen with newer small bore cryoprobes and cryoablation carries very low complication rates. Bleeding through fracture of the tissue around the cryoprobe tract remains the most serious, albeit rare, complication.

Summary

RFA is a particular form of radiofrequency electrosurgery that takes advantage of the ability of radiofrequency alternating current to create heat in biologic tissue. RFA is used for the destruction of unwanted tissue in many medical specialties including cardiology, urology, thoracic surgery, and oncologic surgery. The ability of radiofrequency current to ablate tissue is variable and greatly depends on the tissue to be ablated and the properties of the tissue in which the target lesion is embedded. Several safety issues need to be considered including potential injuries to the operator and patient as well as safety concerns with regard to the effectiveness of RFA. Many different proprietary systems are currently available and it is important that the user of a particular system is very familiar with its particular properties, use, and application algorithms. Cryoablation essentially is the mirror image of the RFA technology and achieves the same results by freezing the target lesion. It has a slightly different safety profile but requires similar skills and techniques for optimal and safe use.

Summary Take Home Points

1. RFA is a particular form of radiofrequency electrosurgery.
2. It uses high frequency alternating low voltage current to create an electromagnetic field around an active electrode.
3. The effect is heating of the target tissue with the goal of complete destruction of the target through coagulation necrosis.
4. The principle concept is to achieve slow and even deposition of thermal energy throughout the target lesion to at least 50°C.

5. It is important to understand the specific algorithm used by each available proprietary design RFA system to achieve the goal of complete ablation.

6. Major safety issues are dispersive electrode burns, injury to vital organ structures, unintended heat-induced injuries to adjacent organs, and incomplete ablations in oncologic applications.

7. Cryoablation in contrast to RFA uses freezing to destroy target lesions. It uses similar techniques to achieve destruction of target lesions. Bleeding is a rare but potentially serious complication of Cryoablation.

References

1. Rhim H, Dodd 3rd GD. Radiofrequency thermal ablation of liver tumors. J Clin Ultrasound. 1999;27:221–9.
2. Siperstein AE, Gitomirski A. History and technological aspects of radiofrequency thermoablation. Cancer J. 2000;6 Suppl 4:S293–303.
3. Pereira PL, Trybenbach J, Schenk M, Subke J, et al. Radiofrequency ablation: in vivo comparison of four commercially available devices in pig livers. Radiology. 2004; 232:482–90.
4. Chang CK, Handy MP, Smith JM, Recht MH, Welling RE. Radiofrequency ablation of the porcine liver with complete hepatic vascular occlusion. Ann Surg Oncol. 2002; 9:594–8.
5. Livraghi T, Solbiati L, Meloni F, Gazelle S, Halpern EF, Goldberg SN. Treatment of focal liver tumors with percutaneous radio-frequency ablation: complications encountered in a multitcenter study. Radiology. 2003;226:441–51.
6. Curley SA, Rizzo F, Ellis LM, Vaughan JN, Val lone P. Radiofrequency ablation of hepatocellular cancer in 110 patients with cirrhosis. Ann Surg. 2000;232:381–91.
7. Kuvshinoff BW, Ota DM. Radiofrequency ablation of liver tumors: influence of technique and tumor size. Surgery. 2002;132:605–11.
8. Aloia TA, Vauthey JN, Loyer EM, Ribero D, Pawlik TM, Wei SH, Curley SA, Zorzi D, Abdalla EK. Solitary colorectal liver metastasis: resection determines outcome. Arch Surg. 2006;141(5):460–6; discussion 466–7.
9. Pawlik TM, Izzo F, Cohen DS, Morris JS, Curley SA. Combined resection and radiofrequency ablation for advanced hepatic malignancies: results in 172 patients. Ann Surg Oncol. 2003;10:1059–69.

10. Principles and Safety of Microwave Ablation

Ryan Z. Swan and David A. Iannitti

Microwave ablation (MWA) is unique among tissue ablation modalities. MWA and the most commonly used ablation modality, radiofrequency ablation (see Chap. 9), both use electromagnetic (EM) energy; however, MWA uses EM energy with a much higher frequency (shorter wavelength) which dramatically alters the way EM energy travels from generator to patient as well as the way heat is generated within tissue. This fundamental difference in physical properties of EM energy makes MWA a unique and powerful ablation tool with significant differences in ablation characteristics compared to other ablation technologies [1–3]. This chapter focuses on the principles for safe and effective use of MWA in the clinical setting. This chapter does not discuss clinically available MWA systems or outcomes of MWA clinical trials.

Basic Principle

A brief review of the physics of EM energy is necessary to understand the differences between RFA and MWA (see Chap. 2) (Table 10.1). Radiofrequency ablation relies upon alternating current (at RF frequencies of 375–500 KHz) within a closed circuit consisting of a generator, an active electrode, the patient, and large dispersive electrodes. Tissue heating occurs at the area of highest current density (the interface between the ablation electrode and tissue). This is termed *resistive* or *joule heating*. Heat is then conducted outward by conductive heat transfer. Alternatively, MWA relies upon the application of EM energy in the microwave frequency range (915 MHz–9.2 GHz) with a wavelength of only a few centimeters, as compared to the wavelength of RF energy of several meters. This wavelength size is important for applications in

L.S. Feldman et al. (eds.), *The SAGES Manual on the Fundamental Use of Surgical Energy (FUSE)*, DOI 10.1007/978-1-4614-2074-3_10, © Springer Science+Business Media, LLC 2012

Table 10.1. Differences in physical properties of MWA and RFA.

	RFA	MWA
Frequency	375–480 kHz	915 MHz–9.2 GHz
Wavelength in tissue	Meters	Centimeters
Mode of energy transfer	AC current	EM waves
	Requires multiple dispersive electrodes and closed circuit	No circuit required
Primary heating mechanism	Resistive at highest current density (RF probe tip)	Dielectric heating within MW near-field (direct effect of EM waves on water molecules)
Secondary heating mechanism	Conductive heating away from RF probe tip into surrounding tissue	Conductive heating from MW near-field into surrounding tissue

tissue ablation. Energy at RF frequency is unable to travel as an EM wave down the RF electrode, and the vast majority of energy is conducted as alternating current. Conversely, the MW wavelength is proportional to the size of the ablation antenna, allowing the MW energy to travel down the antenna as an EM wave. When the EM wave reaches the end of the transmission lines, the EM wave is "broadcast" outward from the antenna in a spherical fashion establishing an electromagnetic field in the immediately surrounding tissue (Fig. 10.1). There is no current flow in MWA and therefore there is no need for a dispersive electrodes (Fig. 10.2). This near-field represents the unique aspect of MWA, as direct heating is delivered to tissue outside the immediate contact interface [4].

Dielectric Heating

Tissue within the microwave near-field is uniformly heated by a phenomenon termed *dielectric heating*, which is the generation of heat by rapid rotation of natural dipole molecules (i.e., water and hydrophilic molecules) in tissue at MW frequency (Fig. 10.3) [5]. When an MW field is applied to tissue, dipole molecules orient to the electric component of the field. The electric component of the MW field, however, rapidly alternates polarity (at 10^9 times per second), and the dipole molecules must rapidly realign. At MW frequencies, the rotation of the dipole molecules begins to lag behind the EM field oscillations resulting in phase displacement and resistive heating within the entire near-field.

a

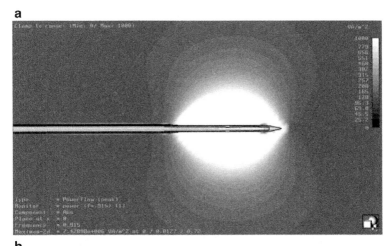

b

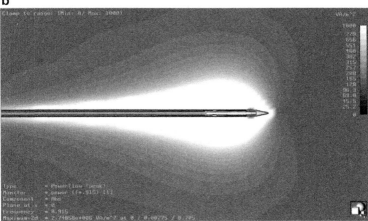

Fig. 10.1. Longitudinal cross-sectional depictions of MW energy being broadcast from (**a**) surgical and (**b**) transcutaneous antennas. Note that the surgical antenna has a round near-field due to the presence of a choke while the transcutaneous antenna has a teardrop-shaped near-field.

Intense and uniform heating occurs within the MW near-field and is conducted outward from the near-field boundary by conductive heat transfer. The effects of an MW near-field on biologic tissue are dependent upon the frequency of the MW energy used as well as the ability of the dipole molecules within the tissue to oscillate within the EM field. This intrinsic tissue property differs between tissue types and is termed the dielectric constant or permittivity.

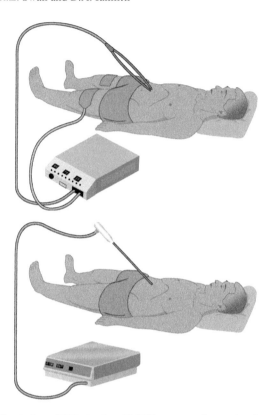

Fig. 10.2. Depiction of RFA (*top*) and MWA systems (*bottom*) and patient. Note the absence of dispersive electrodes (also known as grounding pads) on the patient as MWA does not utilize alternating current flow and does not require a closed circuit as depicted on the patient treated with RFA.

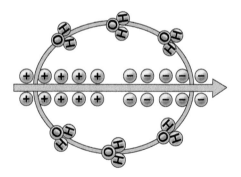

Fig. 10.3. Depiction of dielectric heating. Water molecules, which are natural dipole molecules, rotate within tissues at MW frequency as the EM field changes polarity. Heat is generated by this molecular rotation.

Microwave System Design

Three MW frequency bands (915 MHz, 2.45 GHz, and 9.2 GHz) are currently utilized in commercially available MWA systems, with 915 MHz and 2.45 GHz systems used most frequently for interstitial tissue ablation. Depending on the system design, microwave energy for tissue ablation is generated using either magnetron or semiconductor power amplifiers, the specifics of which will not be discussed here. For practical purposes, however, it should be noted that magnetrons (similar to those used in microwave ovens) are capable of higher energy output and efficiency that requires more sophisticated regulation while transistor-based systems are smaller with more stable power output [4]. Most commercially available MW generators will display power setting (Watts) and ablation time, both of which the user has control over. Most microwave generators do not automatically vary the power output based on tissue temperature or impedance, making for a straightforward display module. Some systems are equipped to monitor tissue temperature via a separate temperature probe that can be inserted near the ablation site. One 915 MHz system will deliver pulses of MW energy to maintain tissue temperature between set limits. Manufacturers of each MWA system will provide recommendations regarding power settings and duration for a given ablation size. Wattage generally ranges from 30 to 180 W and ablation duration ranges from 4 to 10 min depending on the frequency used and system design. Physicians should familiarize themselves with the recommendations for each system, as recommendations vary considerably between systems, and even between different antennas using the same generator.

Both generator types deliver MW energy to the output port where the transmission line is connected. Microwave transmission lines are essentially coaxial cable with an internal conductor, a dielectric layer, and an outer conductor wrapped in an insulating sheath (Fig. 10.4). The MW energy travels as an EM wave from the generator down the transmission line to the ablation hand-piece. The hand-piece is composed of another connector, a handle, and a rigid coaxial transmission line shaft, ending at the radiating tip (antenna) that emits MW energy (Fig. 10.5). The terminology is often confusing: The entire hand-piece is clinically referred to as the antenna, while in bioengineering terms the antenna is actually limited to the radiating tip at the end of the hand-piece. When referring to the *antenna* in this manual, we are referring to the radiating tip at the end of the hand-piece. For purposes of clarity, we will refer to the hand-piece and rigid shaft as the hand-piece.

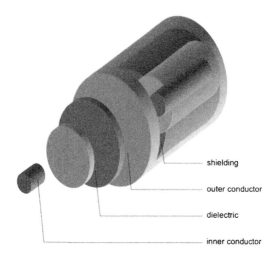

Fig. 10.4. Cross-section of a microwave transmission line. Note the inner conductor, dielectric layer, and outer conductor with insulating sheath.

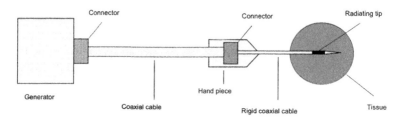

Fig. 10.5. Schematic of a microwave ablation (MWA) system. The microwave generator will generate microwaves at a set frequency which are directed down the flexible transmission line to the hand-piece, which has a connector and a second rigid transmission line ending in the microwave antenna, also called the radiating tip, which is embedded in the target tissue.

The antenna is a portion of the exposed internal conductor of a length calculated to be at least ½ of the MW wavelength when embedded in tissue, with the outer conductor either removed (monopole antenna) or folded back onto itself (dipole antenna). This allows the MW energy to radiate outward from the inner conductor to establish the MW near-field. Various modifications of the basic monopole/dipole antenna design have been implemented to modify the size and shape of the MW near-field (and ablation zone), such as widening the distal inner conductor, adding a distal metal cap, or loading the tip with dielectric material; however, the basic coaxial design remains the same [6]. Microwave transmission lines, hand-piece, and antenna designs vary between manufacturers; however, they can be broadly grouped into surgical and transcutaneous designs based upon their intended use. Transcutaneous MWA hand-pieces are designed to be as minimally invasive as possible (smaller shaft diameter) with longer shafts and built-in cooling systems to prevent abdominal wall burns secondary to shaft heating [7]. Surgical MW hand-pieces are intended for open surgical use and therefore can be of a larger diameter without requiring an internal cooling device to control shaft temperatures.

Impedance Mismatch and Reflected Energy

Each MWA system is specifically designed to optimize delivery of MW energy to tissue; however, there is inherent energy loss in any system due to a phenomenon called *impedance mismatch*. Impedance is the EM equivalent to resistance in an electrical circuit, so higher impedance results in less EM wave transmission. When EM waves travel from one substance with a certain impedance to a second substance with a different impedance, some of the energy will pass through the interface, while some will be reflected back. This is similar to light reflecting off the surface of a lake. Maximum energy deposition will occur when impedance mismatch is minimized. The ablation generator, transmission lines, hand-piece, and antenna are specifically designed to minimize reflected energy and maximize efficient energy deposition into the tissue. This is important in a practical sense because reflected energy can cause significant heating of the ablation hand-piece and transmission lines. For this reason, the microwave generator monitors the reflected energy and will automatically shut off if it reaches a preset thermal and/or reflected energy threshold. Reflected energy secondary to impedance mismatch is also controlled by a mechanism referred to as a choke, which is a metallic ring around the rigid shaft proximal to the radiating tip that is connected to the outer conductor. A choke will create a rounder ablation field by limiting the ability of reflected energy to propagate up the rigid shaft.

Different MWA systems vary significantly in component design, from generator to antenna, and these variations will significantly impact the size and shape of the ablation zone. Even changing from one hand-piece/antenna to another while using the same MW frequency generator can result in a very different ablation. To provide complete tumor ablation and avoid harm to adjacent structures, it is therefore imperative that the user understands that different systems will require different power settings and ablation times to create similar ablation volumes. Clinically available MWA systems undergo extensive preclinical evaluation to establish standardized power and duration settings for a given tissue [8, 9]. The user should, therefore, familiarize themselves with the manufacturer recommendations prior to using an MWA system.

Advantages of MWA

MWA has several advantages over RFA that may translate into higher complete ablation rates. The ability to directly heat tissue within the MW near-field without reliance upon current flow allows for faster and more uniform deposition of energy into the tissue. The reason for this is that MWA does not require strict temperature/impedance control to maintain current flow unlike RFA (see Chap. 9). Microwave energy is directly deposited into tissue within the MW near-field where temperatures can exceed 150°C, as opposed to the controlled range of 60–100°C required during RFA resulting in shorter ablation times for equal volumes. Recommended MWA ablation times vary from 4 to 10 min, depending on the system. Multiple MWA antennas can be powered at the same time, allowing for simultaneous ablation of multiple lesions, again cutting down on overall ablation time. For larger tumors, multiple MWA antennas can also be deployed in an *array* to create a larger ablation zone. Ablation that is not reliant upon current flow is not susceptible to the phenomenon of electric sink, whereby the electric current follows the path of least resistance through the tissue (large blood vessel, bile duct) to the dispersive electrodes, which can result in ablation distortion. Thermal ablation modalities are also subject to convective currents within the target tissue (i.e., perfusion) termed *thermal sink* [10, 11]. Tissue perfusion around a thermal ablation acts like a radiator circulating coolant around an engine, removing heat and thus leading to cooler ablation temperatures and a greater thermal sink effect (Fig. 10.6). The MW near-field does not appear to be effected by perfusion; however, the surrounding zone of conductive heating is affected. The shorter duration and higher temperature gradient generated by MWA result in less perfusion effect in this conductive heating zone compared to RFA [12].

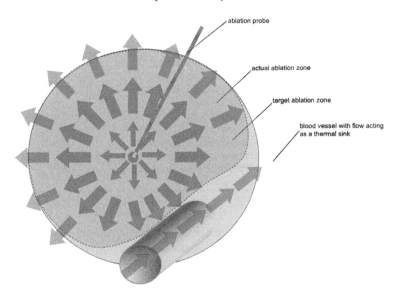

Fig. 10.6. Depiction of thermal sink seen with RFA. When an RF ablation probe is deployed near a large blood vessel, convective heat transfer from the target tissue to the flowing blood will result in ablation zone distortion.

Basic Technique

MWA systems are designed for transcutaneous and surgical use (open and laparoscopic). The choice of MW hand-piece/antenna will be dictated by the approach. Any time the rigid shaft of the hand-piece is to be inserted through the abdominal wall, a transcutaneous hand-piece/antenna should be used to avoid abdominal wall thermal injury.

Operative Microwave Ablation

The location of the target lesion and the condition of the patient will dictate the approach. Certain lesions are more amenable to surgical ablation than percutaneous image-guided ablation, and vice versa. Lesions in close proximity to vital structures or organs should be approached surgically to allow for mobilization to create distance between target lesion and these structures. For hepatic ablation, for example, lesions high on the dome of the liver near the heart and diaphragm or inferior lesions with close proximity to the gallbladder, hepatic flexure of

Table 10.2. Complications of microwave ablation.

Injury	How to prevent injury	Life threatening
Skin burns	Proper spacing (>1.5 cm apart) in parallel and >3 cm between abdominal wall and radiating tip	No
Liver abscess	Perioperative antibiotics	Yes
Liver infarcts	Avoid ablation near portal pedicle	Yes
Vascular fistula	Avoid ablation near portal pedicle	Yes
Bile duct injury	Avoid ablation near portal pedicle	Yes
Hemolysis	Avoid ablation on inferior vena cava	No
Adjacent organ injury	Adequate distance between radiating tip and adjacent organ	Yes

the colon, duodenum, or stomach should be managed surgically. Mobilization of the liver and/or adjacent organs can be performed laparoscopically if the surgeon has this skill set. The insertion of a hand-port is often useful to provide manual traction on the liver when targeting high or posterior lesions. This can both bring the lesion into a more accessible position for targeting and protect the diaphragm/heart/stomach from thermal injury. Insertion of a surgical sponge through a 10–12 mm port or a lap pad through a hand-port to pack between the target lesion and adjacent structures is also a useful technique, as the surgeon cannot leave a hand within the MW near-field during ablation. For hepatic ablation in particular, one should keep in mind that the potential for intra-operative complications is always present and the surgeon should know how to manage major hepatic vascular injury (Table 10.2).

Imaging Guidance

Intra-operative ultrasound (US) is absolutely essential for lesion targeting during MWA. The surgeon should be completely familiar with the operation of the US equipment as well as real-time interpretation of B-mode and color flow Doppler US images. Again, using hepatic ablation as an example, locating the target lesion is often only possible by intra-operative US, and the surgeon can frequently identify additional lesions that may not have been apparent on preoperative cross-sectional imaging. Lesion targeting requires an understanding of the three-dimensional orientation of the lesion in relation to the US probe, as the surgeon must choose the angle by which the ablation antenna will be inserted into the hepatic parenchyma before insertion. Changing antenna direction with the shaft inserted into parenchyma risks causing major vascular or biliary injury. When performing laparoscopic MWA, the surgeon needs to pick not only the angle of approach through the liver parenchyma, but also the angle through the abdominal wall, as the abdominal wall provides little flexibility to change approach angles. A good window to approach hepatic ablation is often in the subxiphoid area.

This three-dimensional spatial orientation becomes very complex when using a flexible laparoscopic US probe that allows for deflection of the US probe to 90° in all directions. Whenever a lesion can be approached with less deflection of the probe, this should be sought in order to simplify the targeting procedure. Targeting a lesion for ablation by US is more or less complex depending on the plane of approach in relation to the US plane. When approaching the lesion *in plane*, with the antenna in line with the US plane, the shaft will appear as a bright white line on the US image. Conversely, when approaching the lesion "out of plane," the shaft will appear as a bright white dot at the point where the shaft crosses the US plane. Approaching a lesion in plane is easier and this approach should be sought if possible unless the surgeon is very comfortable with US targeting.

Positioning of the antenna into the tumor should be performed under real-time US visualization. MWA antennas have an echo-intense metallic puck located at the feed-point where MW energy is emitted that should be positioned in the center of the intended ablation when one antenna is used. When multiple antennas are used to target one lesion, the antennas can be arranged in a triangular array with appropriate spacing around the periphery of the lesion, again under real-time US guidance. The extent of the MWA can be approximated with real-time color flow Doppler US, as the intense activity seen on color flow Doppler closely parallels the zone of coagulation (Fig. 10.7) [13]. This should be done on an intermittent basis, as prolonged placement of the US probe near the MWA zone will cause probe damage.

Percutaneous CT/US Guidance

Lesion location and patient condition can also dictate a percutaneous approach. Caution should be exercised when performing MWA in close proximity to portal pedicles, hepatic veins, or adjacent structures. High-risk patients or patients who have had multiple abdominal operations may benefit from a percutaneous approach if the lesion is in a favorable position. Ablation of locally recurrent disease is also facilitated by a

168   R.Z. Swan and D.A. Iannitti

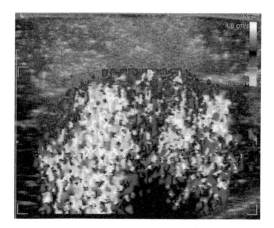

Fig. 10.7. Color flow Doppler imaging during MWA. The boundary of the zone of coagulation closely approximates the intense color flow images obtained during MWA.

percutaneous approach. Cross-sectional imaging (CT) is the usual mode of image guidance for this approach, although US is also used.

Determining Factors of Ablation Size

The final ablation size and shape is determined by multiple factors. The MW energy frequency is a determining factor, with higher frequencies having a shorter wavelength and less penetration into the surrounding tissue. Antenna design will also determine the shape of the MW near-field and thus the ablation zone. Modifications of the antenna (discussed previously, see also Fig 10.1) can affect a more or less spherical near-field. The amount of energy deposited into the near-field is dependent upon the power setting (Watts); therefore, the tissue temperatures in the near-field are also power dependent. With a larger temperature gradient created by higher energy deposition, more conductive heat transfer will occur with less negative effect of "thermal sink" resulting in a larger ablation zone. Similarly, maintaining this steep temperature gradient for a longer duration will result in a larger ablation zone. The practitioner, therefore, can control the shape of the MW near-field by choosing an appropriate ablation antenna and MW frequency, and the final ablation size can be modulated by adjusting Wattage and time. It should also be noted that different tissue types have different permittivity (discussed

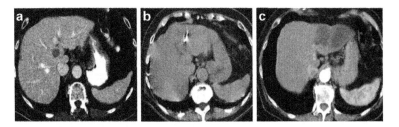

Fig. 10.8. Devascularization of segments II/III from MWA near the portal pedicle. (**a**) Preoperative CT showing a lesion in the caudate lobe of the liver. (**b**) CT-guided percutaneous MWA near the left portal pedicle. (**c**) Post-ablation CT showing devascularization of segments II and III with fluid collections.

previously) which effects the transmission of MW energy and thus the MW near-field and ablation zone. Manufacturers will therefore recommend different power and duration settings for different tissue types.

Safety

Most physicians who use thermal ablation modalities have familiarized themselves with the safe use of RFA, and MWA is often equated with RFA as the two modalities both use EM energy via similar approaches (transcutaneous, laparoscopic, and open surgical ablation) for similar purposes. Significant and potentially dangerous differences in the physical properties of these two thermal ablation systems exist. A thorough understanding of MWA and particularly the differences between MWA and RFA is essential.

The first critical difference between MWA and RFA is that the MW near-field respects no boundary. Practitioners familiar with RFA will understand that creating an air gap between the ablation zone and an organ that needs to be protected will spare that organ from electric current and conductive heating. Microwave, on the other hand, will heat anything within the near-field regardless of the medium surrounding the antenna. An air gap, therefore, will protect an adjacent organ from conductive heat transfer if outside the near-field, but not from direct dielectric heating if inside the near-field. Thermal ablation of adjacent structures can occur if appropriate distance is not maintained. MWA near a portal pedicle can result in devascularization of one or more liver segments (Fig. 10.8) or destruction of bile ducts (Fig. 10.9). Hepatic artery-portal

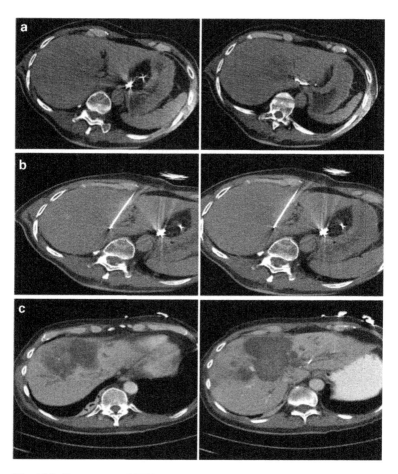

Fig. 10.9. Percutaneous MWA near the portal confluence with subsequent bile duct necrosis. (**a**) Pre-ablation CT showing a lesion near the portal confluence. (**b**) CT-guided MWA of the lesion. (**c**) Post-ablation CT revealing bilateral bile duct necrosis and fluid collections requiring percutaneous trans-hepatic biliary drainage.

vein fistulae have also been seen secondary to ablation near a portal pedicle (Figs. 10.9 and 10.10a). MWA adjacent to hepatic veins can result in hepatic vein thrombosis (Figs. 10.9 and 10.10b) and MWA adjacent to the inferior vena cava can result in hemolysis postoperatively. Adjacent tissue and organs (stomach, gallbladder, colon, kidney, diaphragm) should similarly be protected.

MWA and some RFA systems utilize internal cooling systems; however, the reason that these cooling systems are employed is very

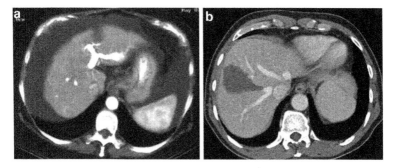

Fig. 10.10. Complications of peri-vascular ablation. (**a**) Post-ablation arterial phase CT revealing a hepatic artery to portal vein fistula requiring angiographic embolization. (**b**) Post-ablation venous phase CT revealing right hepatic vein thrombosis requiring anticoagulation.

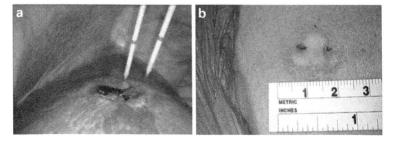

Fig. 10.11. Transcutaneous MWA resulting in skin burn. (**a**) Multi-antenna MWA of a hepatic lesion. (**b**) Skin burn requiring full-thickness excision.

different between modalities. In RFA, internal cooling systems are used to maintain a constant probe temperature for optimal tissue temperature/impedance to maintain current flow. Internal cooling systems in transcutaneous MWA systems are used to avoid heating of the hand-piece and transmission lines due to reflected energy. Heating of the rigid shaft of the hand-piece when used in a transcutaneous fashion can result in full thickness abdominal wall burns (Fig. 10.11). The risk is particularly high when multiple antennas are used in a closely arranged array [14]. The reflected energy that causes shaft heating can be amplified if the antennae are placed too closely together or not in parallel; hence, one manufacturer recommends a minimum spacing distance of 1.5 cm and provides a plastic antenna spacer to maintain spacing and a parallel orientation. Additionally, a minimum of 3 cm should be maintained between radiating tip of the ablation shaft and the abdominal wall [14].

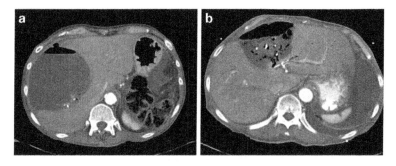

Fig. 10.12. Post-ablation intra-hepatic fluid collection vs. intra-hepatic abscess. (**a**) Post-ablation CT showing intra-hepatic fluid collection with air-fluid level without infection that resolved without intervention. (**b**) Post-ablation CT showing an intra-hepatic abscess with clinical and radiographic signs of infection requiring percutaneous intervention.

All thermal ablation modalities create a zone of coagulative necrosis, and this necrotic material is at risk for infection. Post-ablation abscess formation is a rare but significant occurrence. Perioperative antibiotics to cover skin and enteric flora should be administered preoperatively and continued for 24 h. A longer course of antibiotics should be considered if the biliary tree is contaminated. Initial post-ablation imaging (at 2–4 weeks) will often reveal intrahepatic fluid collections containing air fluid levels as a result of the MWA induced tissue necrosis. These "cold" abscesses will resolve spontaneously over time. They can usually be differentiated from a post-ablation abscess by the patients' clinical course and the characteristics of the fluid collection (Fig. 10.12).

Oncologic Safely

Thermal ablation modalities are increasingly utilized for a wide range of primary and metastatic malignancies in many tissue types. MWA has the potential to increase complete ablation rates and decrease local recurrence compared to RFA. Single center studies have demonstrated significant improvements in ablation success and local recurrence [15]; however, a prospective randomized trial to compare these two modalities has yet to be performed. Appropriate MW generator/frequency and antenna selection, power and time settings based on manufacturer recommendations, and optimal image-guided antenna positioning can result in exceptional complete ablation rates with minimal morbidity.

Summary

MWA is a form of thermal ablation that utilizes electromagnetic waves to establish a microwave near-field where direct tissue heating occurs by a phenomenon called "dielectric heating." MWA does not rely upon electric current and is not subject to the limitations that electric current imposes. The shape of the MW near-field is determined by MW frequency and antenna design whereas the amount of energy deposited into the near-field and the final ablation size is determined by the power and duration of ablation as well as the type of tissue being targeted. Compared to current-dependent thermal ablation modalities MWA does not appear to be as sensitive to thermal sink due to higher temperatures and shorter ablation times. The user should be familiar with manufacturer recommendations for ablation settings for the MWA equipment that they have selected. The user should also be aware of significant differences in safety precautions between MWA and RFA when using MWA equipment. When used appropriately, MWA can provide exceptional complete ablation rates with minimal morbidity for a wide range of primary and metastatic lesions.

Take Home Points

1. MWA is a form of thermal ablation that utilizes electromagnetic waves rather than electrical current.
2. Direct heating of tissue around the microwave antenna occurs by causing polarized molecules in the tissue to rotate extremely rapidly resulting in the generation of heat.
3. MWA allows for higher tissue temperatures and faster ablation times compared to radiofrequency ablation because MWA does not require controlled tissue impedance to maintain current flow.
4. It is absolutely essential that the user of an MWA system become familiar with the recommended power and time settings for that system before use.
5. Image-guided antenna positioning is essential to avoid complication and obtain complete ablation of the target lesion.
6. Major differences in the physical properties of microwave and radiofrequency ablation exist, and the user should be familiar with safe techniques for MWA to avoid potentially serious complications.

References

1. Ahmed M, Brace CL, Lee Jr FT, Goldberg SN. Principles of and advances in percutaneous ablation. Radiology. 2011;258(2):351–69.
2. Padma S, Martinie JB, Iannitti DA. Liver tumor ablation: percutaneous and open approaches. J Surg Oncol. 2009;100(8):619–34.
3. Bhardwaj N, Strickland AD, Ahmad F, Dennison AR, Lloyd DM. Liver ablation techniques: a review. Surg Endosc. 2010;24(2):254–65.
4. Brace CL. Microwave tissue ablation: biophysics, technology, and applications. Crit Rev Biomed Eng. 2010;38(1):65–78.
5. Gabriel C, Gabriel S, Grant EH, Halstead BSJ, Mingos DMP. Dielectric parameters relevant to microwave dielectric heating. Chem Soc Rev. 1998;27:213–24.
6. Bertram JM, Yang D, Converse MC, Webster JG, Mahvi DM. Antenna design for microwave hepatic ablation using an axisymmetric electromagnetic model. Biomed Eng Online. 2006;5:15.
7. Sindram D, Haley K, McKillop IH, Martinie JB, Iannitti DA. Determination of angle, depth and distance of antennae as skin burn risks in microwave ablation in a porcine model. J Int Oncol. 2010;3(1):46–52.
8. Hope WW, Schmelzer TM, Newcomb WL, et al. Guidelines for power and time variables for microwave ablation in a porcine liver. J Gastrointest Surg. 2008;12(3):463–7.
9. Hope WW, Schmelzer TM, Newcomb WL, et al. Guidelines for power and time variables for microwave ablation in an in vivo porcine kidney. J Surg Res. 2009; 153(2):263–7.
10. Lu DS, Raman SS, Limanond P, et al. Influence of large peritumoral vessels on outcome of radiofrequency ablation of liver tumors. J Vasc Interv Radiol. 2003;14(10): 1267–74.
11. Patterson EJ, Scudamore CH, Owen DA, Nagy AG, Buczkowski AK. Radiofrequency ablation of porcine liver in vivo: effects of blood flow and treatment time on lesion size. Ann Surg. 1998;227(4):559–65.
12. Wright AS, Sampson LA, Warner TF, Mahvi DM, Lee Jr FT. Radiofrequency versus microwave ablation in a hepatic porcine model. Radiology. 2005;236(1):132–9.
13. Byrd JF, Agee N, McKillop IH, Sindram D, Martinie JB, Iannitti DA. Colour doppler ultrasonography provides real-time microwave field visualisation in an ex vivo porcine model. HPB (Oxford). 2011;13(6):400–3.
14. Sindram D, Haley K, McKillop IH, Martinie JB, Iannitti DA. Determination of angle, depth, and distance of antennae as skin burn risks in microwave ablation in a porcine model. J Intervent Oncol. 2010;3(1):46–52.
15. Martin RC, Scoggins CR, McMasters KM. Safety and efficacy of microwave ablation of hepatic tumors: a prospective review of a 5-year experience. Ann Surg Oncol. 2010;17(1):171–8.

11. Surgical Energy Systems in Pediatric Surgery

Gretchen Purcell Jackson

Pediatric patients have unique anatomic and physiologic characteristics that must be considered when using energy devices. Although most general surgeons may never operate on infants or children, they are likely to encounter patients with alterations in body composition that pose similar challenges. Such patients might include amputees, individuals with multiple prostheses or implanted devices, cachectic cancer patients, or severely edematous individuals. This chapter presents the distinguishing features of pediatric patients and their implications for the use of energy devices.

Anatomic and Physiologic Considerations in Infants and Children

Compared with adults, infants and children have a greater body surface area to volume ratio, but less total body surface area [1, 2]. High-resistance tissues are often located in close proximity to areas of low resistance, and the path for current flow may be even less predictable in children than it is in adults. The limited surface area must accommodate the surgical site, all monitoring devices, and dispersive electrodes, making overlap or compromise of such devices more likely. Newborns are particularly at risk for injury from drainage of sterile preparation, irrigation, or body fluids, especially when a dispersive electrode is placed below an abdominal operative site. Such fluids can cause burns by interfering with the contact between the patient's skin and a dispersive electrode or by creating aberrant current pathways through wetting of the sheets between the patient and the operative table [3, 4]. Because of the small size of a pediatric patient, any injury can be catastrophic.

L.S. Feldman et al. (eds.), *The SAGES Manual on the Fundamental Use of Surgical Energy (FUSE)*, DOI 10.1007/978-1-4614-2074-3_11,
© Springer Science+Business Media, LLC 2012

Current flow is greatest in tissues of high water content, and children, especially newborns, have significantly more total body water, making the tissues low resistance and good conductors of current. Newborn infants have an excess of total body water, primarily in the form of extracellular fluid, which is typically lost during the first week of life. Whereas adult patients are approximately 60% water, term infants are composed of approximately 75% water. Infants who are preterm or small for gestational age have even higher proportions of total body water. For example, an infant born at 23 weeks' gestational age is approximately 90% water [2]. When these infants require surgery, the high water content of the tissues can rapidly conduct or concentrate energy. Water content reaches adult levels at the age of approximately 18 months [1].

Smaller anatomic structures require smaller instruments, both of which may concentrate current in critical areas. Thermal burns have been reported at the site of miniature electrocardiogram electrodes because the small size of the electrodes resulted in a high current density despite the use of low power settings [5]. Small diameter airways found in children are also at particular risk for operative fires because they combine combustible materials and an oxygen-rich environment in a confined space. Although oropharyngeal procedures such as tonsillectomy can be conducted safely in children using electrosurgical techniques [6], several precautions can reduce the risk of fire. Ideally, an endotracheal tube cuff can separate the upper and lower airways. For younger children, an appropriate-sized, uncuffed endotracheal tube should be employed to avoid a large air leak that could increase nitrous oxide or oxygen concentrations at the operative site. If the patient has comorbid cardiac or pulmonary conditions that require a high concentration of oxygen, the surgeon might want to avoid an electrosurgical device, especially if set to the modulated and high-voltage *coagulation* waveform, which is prone to sparking [7].

Electrosurgical Unit Outputs in Children

Electrosurgical systems all have distinctive properties including different output waveforms, safety features, and device compatibilities, and it is imperative to review manufacturer specifications and recommendations to operate safely any particular unit, especially in the pediatric population (see Chaps. 2 and 3) [8]. For all patients, the lowest possible power settings that achieve the desired thermal effect should be used, but in children, the maximal settings employed are generally much lower than those used in adults. Many pediatric surgeons seldom use power settings greater than 12 W even in adolescents, and they limit power settings in all modes to 8–10 W in newborns.

Safe settings may vary by manufacturer or *even across individual devices*, and a biomedical engineer may need to calibrate each generator individually. For example, one manufacturer provides the following instructions for its neonatal dispersive electrodes, which are intended for use for preterm infants weighing 450–2,700 g:

> "Prior to initial pad use, the electrosurgical generator should be calibrated by a qualified biomedical engineer or technician to determine the control setting that represents the maximum current level (300 mA) recommended for this return electrode. A standard electrosurgical analyzer that uses a 125 Ω load should be used for this calibration. A reading of 300 mA should be identified in each cut, coag, and blend mode."

This company recommends that each unit is calibrated and then labeled with maximal power settings for neonatal patients with a sticker. Surgeons should routinely check the settings of all electrosurgical units prior to starting a procedure, especially if the operating room equipment is used for patients of varied ages and sizes.

Dispersive Electrodes in Children

Dispersive electrodes are available in weight-based sizes for infants and children, usually in neonatal, pediatric, and adult forms. The weight limits will vary by manufacturer, but in general, the lower limit of weight is approximately 400 g or 1 lb. Adult dispersive electrodes are used when patient's weight exceeds approximately 30 lb or 13.6 kg.

The guidelines for positioning of dispersive electrodes are the same for adults and children, but the small size and proximity of structures in pediatric patients make placement more challenging. The ideal site will be convex in shape, close to the surgical site, and over a well-vascularized muscle mass, but remote from scar tissue, bony structures, or excessive adipose tissue. In a neonate, the best site is on the back between the scapulae and sacrum, but this location is at risk for compromise from pooling of fluids—either from skin preparation, drainage from operative sites, or irrigation during a procedure. In very small babies, almost any site is at risk. In older or larger infants, dispersive electrodes can be positioned on the back, torso, or thigh [8].

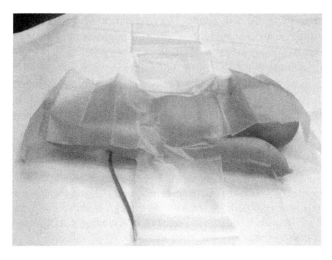

Fig. 11.1. A depiction of a newborn with the dispersive electrode protected by fluid-resistant adhesive drapes.

Some surgeons protect the site of dispersive electrodes with fluid-resistant adhesive drapes as shown in Fig. 11.1. These drapes can also help keep an infant warm during the surgical procedures. The neonatal skin is extremely fragile, so care must be taken when adhesive on the drapes or electrodes are removed from the infant. As with all patients, the dispersive electrode should *never* be cut or modified to fit the patient. The electrode edges should not be allowed to overlap, and they must not contact other patient leads or monitoring devices. When possible, pediatric surgeons should consider use of bipolar devices to avoid the risks associated with the dispersive electrode and the inclusion of the patient in the electrical circuit.

Electrosurgery in Pregnancy

Surgical interventions such as appendectomy or cholecystectomy are sometimes necessary for pregnant women. There is no evidence to suggest that electrosurgery in a pregnant mother poses risk to the fetus at any point during gestation. The electrolyte-rich amniotic fluid protects the fetus from concentration of current, and the output frequency of electrosurgical generators is above the level that stimulates muscle contraction for both the adult patient and fetus. The only risk to the fetus during a delivery or prenatal intervention would be direct contact between an active electrode and the fetus, which could produce thermal injury [9].

Summary

Most energy devices can be used safely in pediatric patients, but surgeons must be aware of the unique anatomic and physiologic considerations that affect their use. Smaller anatomic structures and pediatric instruments can concentrate current, and the proximity of low- and high-resistance tissues, monitoring devices, and surgical instruments can lead to unpredictable electrical pathways. The variations seen in patients provide an excellent model for thinking about energy-device safety in any patient with altered body composition.

References

1. Holcomb III GW, Murphy JP, editors. Ashcraft's pediatric surgery. 5th ed. Philadelphia: Saunders; 2010.
2. Ambalavanan N. Fluid, electrolyte, and nutrition management of the newborn. Medscape Reference. New York: WebMD; 2010.
3. Demir E, O'Dey DM, Pallua N. Accidental burns during surgery. J Burn Care Res. 2006;27:895–900.
4. Masuko K, Ichiyanagi K. Still another mode of electrosurgical burn: a report of two cases and an experiment. Anesth Analg. 1973;52:19–22.
5. Finlay B, Couchie D, Boyce L, Spencer E. Electrosurgery burns resulting from use of miniature ECG electrodes. Anesthesiology. 1974;41:263–9.
6. Maddern BR. Electrosurgery for tonsillectomy. Laryngoscope. 2002;112:11–3.
7. Mattucci KF, Militana CJ. The prevention of fire during oropharyngeal electrosurgery. Ear Nose Throat J. 2003;82:107–9.
8. Dennis V. Keeping pediatric patients safe during electrosurgery. OR Nurse. 2011;5:48.
9. Soderstrom R. Principles of electrosurgery as applied to gynecology. In: Rock J, Jones H, editors. Te Linde's operative gynecology. 9th ed. Philadelphia: Lippincott Williams & Wilkins; 2003.

12. Integration of Energy Systems with Other Medical Devices

Stephanie B. Jones and Marc A. Rozner

Electromagnetic interference (EMI) from medical equipment may originate from multiple sources and interfere with implantable electronic devices in the patient [1]. Such implanted devices include cardiac implantable electronic devices (CIED), i.e., pacemakers and implantable defibrillators; deep brain, spinal cord, vagal nerve and sacral nerve (bladder) stimulators; implantable infusion pumps and cochlear implants. The scope of this discussion is limited to CIED.

It is estimated that over three million patients are currently treated with conventional pacemakers for bradycardia pacing, and approximately 750,000 are implanted in the United States yearly, according to industry sources. Greater than 300,000 patients have implanted defibrillators (ICD), which provide high-voltage therapy for ventricular tachycardia/fibrillation as well as conventional pacing for bradycardia. The Heart Rhythm Society estimates that more than 10,000 ICDs are implanted per month, with an expected prevalence of 670,000 by 2020. Many of the CIEDs, whether or not high-voltage therapy is present, have a pacing lead designed to activate the left ventricle (called cardiac resynchronization therapy (CRT) or biventricular (BiV) pacing) for the patient who has significant cardiomyopathy.

EMI can be generated by many devices in the operating room and elsewhere within the hospital. These include monopolar electrosurgical and endoscopic devices, radiofrequency ablation (RFA) systems, electrocardiographic monitors, fluid and blood warmers, MRI and CT scanners, and peripheral nerve stimulators. Ultrasonic shears generate mechanical rather than electromagnetic energy and are therefore safe to use in the presence of implantable devices. One must remember, however, that any energy device has the potential to cause damage, particularly to surrounding structures (Fig. 12.1).

Multiple factors determine the effects of EMI on CIED, which include the distance between the energy source and CIED leads and how the

L.S. Feldman et al. (eds.), *The SAGES Manual on the Fundamental Use of Surgical Energy (FUSE)*, DOI 10.1007/978-1-4614-2074-3_12, © Springer Science+Business Media, LLC 2012

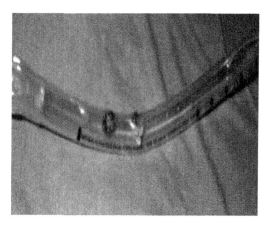

Fig. 12.1. Any energy device has the potential to cause damage, particularly to surrounding structures. Shown here is a endotracheal tube damaged by an ultrasonic energy device. (From Balakrishnan and Kuriakose [15], with permission of Lippincott Williams & Wilkins).

CIED leads are oriented relative to the generated EMI. For any given energy source, intensity, frequency, and waveform of the generated signal all contribute to the EMI. In addition, EMI might induce unusual effects on a poorly functioning or malfunctioning device, which might otherwise cause no symptoms in the ambulatory patient [2, 3].

Although more recent CIED technology has improved shielding against EMI effects, potential for interference with CIED function, damage to the device, or injury to the patient does exist. Most commonly, inappropriate inhibition or triggering of a pacemaker or ICD may occur if the device interprets EMI as a cardiac signal. Although the most common effect results in pacing inhibition, an ICD can deliver high-voltage therapy if the device interprets EMI as a ventricular arrhythmia. Less commonly, noise detection may result in unintended asynchronous pacing or failure to detect a ventricular arrhythmia. Actual spurious reprogramming of a current-model CIED is nearly impossible, but electrical resets to default and safety modes certainly take place.

EMI may damage the electrical components of CIED or cause a thermal injury where the lead enters the endocardium. Such tissue damage can raise pacing thresholds (Fig. 12.2). The electrical signal can also be conducted by the CIED lead, inducing a cardiac arrhythmia such as atrial or ventricular fibrillation.

Certain attributes of the CIED itself will influence its potential to be affected by EMI. The number of leads and possibly their configuration

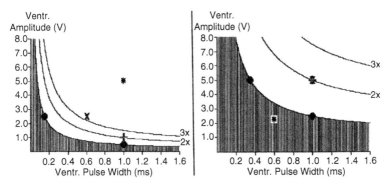

Fig. 12.2. Preoperative (*left panel*) and postoperative (*right panel*) "strength-duration" plots of pacing output and capture thresholds from an 82.5 kg, 48-year-old woman with hypertrophic obstructive cardiomyopathy who underwent a paraspinous sarcoma excision in the prone position, where both standard monopolar and argon beam devices were used and who had a one blood volume (5.5 L) transfusion. In a strength-duration plot, any combination of pacing pulse amplitude and width in the non-shaded area would be expected to provide ventricular capture. In the *left panel*, the "+" (1.5 V, 1.0 ms) was the recommended setting by the programmer to conserve battery energy, the "*X*" (2.5 V, 0.6 ms) was the presenting output, and the "*" (5 V, 1.0 ms) was the setting upon presentation to the operating room. In the *right panel*, the pacing threshold has increased several-fold, likely due to effects from EMI and the volume resuscitation. The "+" and the "*X*" (recommended pacing output and the current output—5 V, 1.0 ms) overlie each other. The "*" (2.5 V, 0.6 ms) was the initial presenting output and is now clearly inadequate. (Courtesy of M. Rozner, PhD, MD, Houston, TX).

[4] is an obvious factor, as more wiring in the heart increases the surface area available to detect EMI. Thus, dual chamber pacemakers (Fig. 12.3) are more likely than single chamber pacemakers to have problems with EMI. The distance between anode and cathode is also relevant. In a unipolar lead, the anode is the pacemaker case itself, with the cathode at the tip of the lead. This creates more lead distance over which electrical signal may be detected. By contrast, a bipolar lead tip contains both anode and cathode, creating a very small electrically active area. Fortunately, the majority of current pacemakers and all ICDs utilize bipolar sensing leads.

When conducting a preoperative evaluation of a patient with an existing CIED, a standard approach should be used. Much of the information presented below has been derived from the American Society of Anesthesiologists (ASA) Practice Advisory for the Perioperative

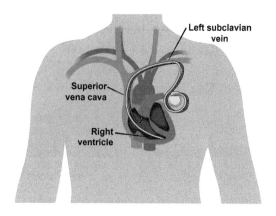

Fig. 12.3. Dual chamber pacemaker.

Management of Patients with CIED: Pacemakers and Implantable Cardioverter-Defibrillators [5] and the Consensus Statement from the Heart Rhythm Society [6]. It should be kept in mind that both of these documents represent practice advisories and expert opinion; neither is a guideline, indicating an insufficient number of adequately controlled studies on which to base recommendations.

First, one needs to determine if the patient has a CIED. Although this may seem obvious, such information may be missed when preparing a patient for an urgent or emergent procedure. A thorough history and physical exam will help verify the presence of a pacemaker or ICD generator and the indication for device placement. The determination of pacing dependence (which could be present in any CIED patient) as well as the presence of a high-voltage device (ICD) serves to identify those patients who will have the greatest potential for harm from typical EMI effects. Absolute pacing dependence refers to the patient who has no underlying ventricular systoles, owing to either sinoatrial or atrioventricular nodal disease. Functional pacing dependence refers to the patient who will suffer hemodynamic embarrassment at any system failure to sense/pace the myocardium in an optimal fashion.

Ideally, the patient will have an identification card on hand in order to easily establish the type of device. In the absence of such, a chest X-ray can reveal identifying codes [7]. If surgical urgency allows for more investigative time, medical records pertaining to CIED placement, function and evaluation should be obtained. Without these records or a reliable history from the patient, it may not be possible to ascertain whether the patient is fully dependent upon pacing function. In that case, the CIED can be reprogrammed to its minimal pacing rate to reveal the patient's native rate and rhythm. In most settings, this will require the assistance of a pacing service or a manufacturer's representative. Finally, the device should be fully evaluated for appropriate programming and function by a qualified physician. Again, if time does not permit this, an electrocardiogram might be helpful to identify pacing and sensing issues.

Next, the likelihood of EMI occurrence should be determined. It should be understood that the overall effects of EMI are highly variable with different CIED models. Consequently, the ideal preventative strategy would be avoiding the use of EMI generating devices altogether in the presence of CIED. Bipolar electrosurgical devices and ultrasonic instruments may be options, although this is largely dependent upon the nature of the surgical procedure. Of note, there is a lack of evidence establishing superiority of bipolar over monopolar electrosurgical instruments in preventing EMI. With bipolar instruments, the electrical current simply travels between the much smaller tissue volume that is contained between the two electrodes of the bipolar instrument compared with the current path inherent to monopolar instrumentation, which extends from the handheld instrument containing the active electrode to a dispersive electrode located remotely on the patient. Therefore, while bipolar instrumentation generally provides a measure of safety when used at a distance from the CIED, a bipolar RF instrument may potentially cause interference if used in close proximity to the device.

If use of a monopolar electrosurgical device is deemed necessary, attention should be paid to its settings. The continuous, low-voltage sinusoidal waveform of the "cut" mode creates the least interference with CIED when compared to that associated with the modulated outputs of the "coagulation" and "blend" modes [8]. The relatively low voltage and sustained continuous output of the "cut" waveform as generally used has a peak amplitude less than 2,000 V, which creates an electromagnetic field that is easily filtered by the CIED. On the other hand, the modulated and high-voltage "coagulation" waveforms are characterized by low duty cycles (typically about 6%) and high peak-to-peak voltages that may reach 10,000 V. Such intermittent high-voltage outputs can create broad spectrum electromagnetic "noise" that is more difficult to filter. With either mode (monopolar or bipolar), the lowest possible ESU power setting that achieves the desired surgical effect should be selected, and short, intermittent bursts of low-voltage output are preferred over the use of modulated outputs such as "coag" and "blend." Open circuit activation is also associated with the generation of increased capacitance in the

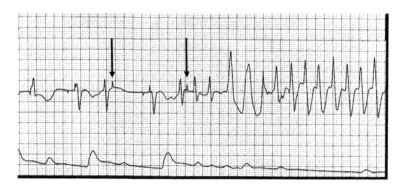

Fig. 12.4. Ventricular tachycardia caused by R-on-T phenomenon. *Arrows* indicate pacemaker spikes. (From Rozner [16], with permission of Elsevier).

entire circuit, and may contribute to an increased risk of CIED interference. Consequently the ESU should be activated only when the electrosurgical instrument is in contact with patient tissue.

Reprogramming of pacing parameters to an asynchronous mode (DOO, AOO, VOO) is often recommended to avoid pacemaker inhibition when EMI is erroneously detected as native cardiac signal. However, this is not without risk, due to the possibility of R-on-T phenomenon inducing a ventricular arrhythmia (Fig. 12.4) (Table 12.1). Asynchronous modes should probably be avoided in patients prone to ventricular tachycardia or ventricular fibrillation.

Some pacemakers have rate-adaptive functions, intended to mimic physiologic heart rate alterations during exercise or sleep. Most practitioners recommended suspension of these rate-adaptive functions, as activities such as surgical preparation or mechanical ventilation can precipitate increases in pacing rate, which can be misinterpreted, leading to improper and injurious treatment [9].

If an ICD is present, consideration should be given to suspension of antitachyarrhythmia functions. Defibrillation and temporary pacing equipment must be immediately available during this time and until these functions have been fully reestablished in the postoperative period. ICD function should ideally be suspended via reprogramming. Several authorities now suggest that magnet placement on an ICD to suspend antitachyarrhythmia therapy might be acceptable provided that magnet function has been verified preoperatively, the patient will be positioned such that the magnet placement will be continuously observable, the magnet will not interfere with surgery, and magnet

Table 12.1. NBG (North American society of pacing and electrophysiology/British pacing and electrophysiology group) generic pacemaker codes.

Chamber(s) paced	Chamber(s) sensed	Response to sensing	Programmability, rate modulation	Multisite pacing
O = none	O = none	O = none	O = none	O = none
A = atrium	A = atrium	T = triggered	R = rate modulation	A = atrium
V = ventricle	V = ventricle	I = inhibited		V = ventricle
D = dual	D = dual	D = dual		D = dual

Adapted from Bernstein et al. [7], with permission of Wiley

188   S.B. Jones and M.A. Rozner

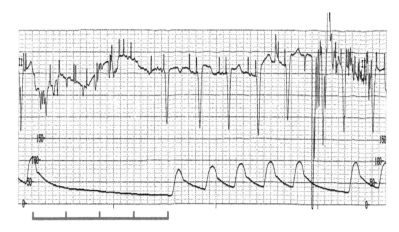

Fig. 12.5. Inhibition of pacemaker by EMI. Top line is EKG, bottom is arterial waveform. Note complete inhibition of pacemaker rhythm and lack of perfusion during the period denoted by the *red line*. The failure of mechanical systoles would not be readily apparent if monitoring EKG alone. (Figure courtesy of M. Rozner, PhD, MD, Houston, TX).

placement will not likely injure the patient. Although a magnet will usually disable antitachyarrhythmia functions of ICD devices, it typically will not alter any pacing functions present within the device. Furthermore, if monopolar electrosurgery is used during the case, the device should be interrogated postoperatively. Most ICDs will spontaneously resume antitachyarrhythmia functions upon removal of the magnet, but an occasional model will be permanently disabled until actively reprogrammed. However, an ICD might not deliver high-voltage therapy even in the presence of VT if the VT rate or morphology does not meet preprogrammed criteria.

Placing a magnet on a conventional pacemaker frequently results in conversion to an asynchronous pacing mode, although this effect might vary depending upon programming. The result of magnet placement may also be affected by remaining battery life of the device. Due to the unpredictability of magnet effect on pacemaker function, interrogation of the device preoperatively are preferred in all but emergency circumstances.

Once in the operating room, intraoperative ASA standards dictate electrocardiographic monitoring [10]. However, the EKG signal often will display interference from EMI and be unhelpful in detecting alteration of pacemaker function. Thus, a perfusion monitor, either a pulse oximetry plethysmograph or invasive arterial waveform (Fig. 12.5)

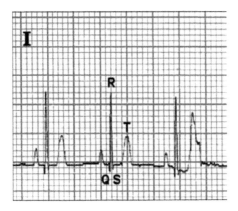

Fig. 12.6. Spurious ST elevation created by EMI. (Adapted from De Marco and Maggi [12], with permission).

should be utilized as well [6, 11]. ST segment monitoring may also be compromised by EMI. This should be kept in mind when caring for patients at risk for perioperative cardiac ischemia (Fig. 12.6) [12].

For monopolar instrumentation, EMI can be minimized with careful attention to appropriate positioning of the dispersive electrode relative to the location of the CIED generator, leads, and the surgical site. Where possible, the dispersive electrode should be positioned such that the presumed current path does not cross the CIED system (Fig. 12.7). Positioning may require some creativity when surgery is performed superior to the umbilicus in a patient with a CIED generator implanted at the infraclavicular position, the most commonly used site today. For example, for surgical procedures on the breast ipsilateral to the CIED, the dispersion pad may be most appropriately placed on the same side arm. For the patient with an unusual system configuration (e.g., an abdominal generator implant with leads tunneled to an infraclavicular location for entry into a subclavian vein), the dispersive electrode might be best placed on a site that is 180° from the surgical site in an axial direction, since presumed current flow perpendicular to the lead configuration will produce less EMI than flow parallel to the leads. A second goal is to keep the current path as far away from the CIED as possible.

When applying RF electrical current by way of an instrument (i.e., a forceps or hemostat) or the hand instrument is not in contact with patient

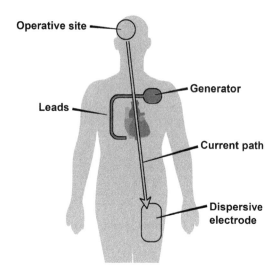

Fig. 12.7. Illustration of undesired electrosurgical current path crossing the CIED system. (Original illustration courtesy of Mark Trankina, MD, Birmingham, AL).

tissue, a capacitor is created which increases the risk of EMI. An additional mechanism for the creation of EMI relates to the fact that the arcing (active electrode not in direct contact with the tissues) actually demodulates the frequency of the electrosurgical current, defeating the existing CIED electrical filtering system.

Similar principles should be employed when performing coagulation and desiccation of large volumes of tissue that is a characteristic of RFA. The CIED should be kept out of the current path, and contact between the pulse generator and leads should be avoided. Patients in whom RFA is chosen as an alternative to surgery due to significant comorbid conditions likely have a higher prevalence of CIED than average. In one study published by Skonieczki in the *European Journal of Radiology*, fifteen percutaneous RFA procedures were performed in patients with CIED. One device was found to have been reprogrammed from VOO to VVI mode (which likely represents an electrical reset), with no inhibition noted, and another showed four episodes of pacemaker inhibition and increased atrial rate, although this effect was believed to be clinically insignificant [13]. No damage to CIED was revealed by postprocedure interrogation, and the authors concluded that RFA could be safely performed in these patients with appropriate perioperative

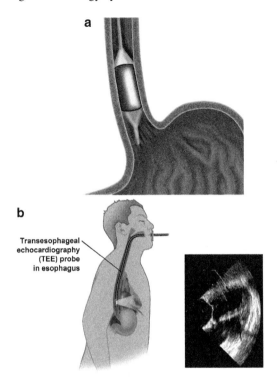

Fig. 12.8. (**a**, **b**) Comparison of placement of a circumferential ablation catheter for treatment of Barrett's esophagus with that of a transesophageal echocardiography probe. Note proximity to heart and therefore any CIED that may be present.

planning. However, in some circumstances, an electrical reset can require replacement of the generator.

Endoscopic devices employ EMI emitting energy sources as well. For lower gastrointestinal procedures, this is probably of lesser concern. However, for procedures occurring in the esophagus or stomach or possbily the transverse colon, one needs to be mindful of the presence of CIED (Fig. 12.8). Stretta, a proprietary device used to treat gastroesophageal reflux, is a monopolar device. The BARRX device, an instrument used in the treatment of Barrett's esophagus, is bipolar, but during the procedure the electrodes are in very close proximity to the heart. Even more worrisome, such procedures may be taking place in busy free-standing endoscopy centers with little in the way of cardiology resources should an untoward event occur. The physicians' manual for these devices should be consulted for CIED recommendations.

In general, all CIEDs should be interrogated in the postoperative period when electrosurgical devices have been utilized. The timing of this posotoperative evaluation will depend upon the proximity of the EMI to the CIED system, whether or not the CIED was reprogrammed for the procedure, and the nature of the surgery. The preoperative CIED evaluation should identify the appropriate timing of the postoperative interrogation [17]. This is to ascertain any changes in settings or cardiac response to those settings, and to restore functionality, if necessary. One caveat is that endocardial damage causing an increase in the pacing threshold may not be apparent for up to 24–48 h.

Opinions do differ on the degree of attention that should be paid to CIED. Cheng et al. studied 92 patients with CIED undergoing a variety of procedures [14]. One ICD tripped its elective replacement indicator; no other changes were detected. The authors suggest that special measures are not needed so long as the EMI is not in close proximity to CIED. However, given the robust shielding systems present in current CIED, the sample size of 92 may simply be too small to detect a significant number of complications. The authors do agree that postprocedural evaluation of CIED should be performed.

Important points:

- Does the patient have a CIED? Is it an ICD or pacemaker? What is the indication for the device and what are the settings? Is the patient pacing dependent?
- Is an electrosurgical device needed for the procedure? If so, the current path should not cross the CIED, a continuous low-voltage waveform (pure "cut") mode should be used if possible, with short, intermittent bursts at the lowest power settings possible.
- Interrogate all devices postoperatively to ensure return to preoperative settings and function. Note that for some patients and some operations, the pacing rate might need to be increased to provide appropriate cardiac output and expected oxygen delivery.
- Be aware of CIED in nonoperating room locales such as the endoscopy and radiology suites. The increasing use of RF electrosurgical devices in these settings, including those designed for RFA, can pose a potential additional risk if the entire procedural team is not aware of the CIED implications.

References

1. Madigan JD, Choudhri AF, Chen J, Spotnitz HM, Oz MC, Edwards N. Surgical management of the patient with an implanted cardiac device: implications of electromagnetic interference. Ann Surg. 1999;230(5):639–47.
2. Boriani G, Biffi M, Martignani C. Uneventful right ventricular perforation with displacement of a pacing lead into the left thorax. J Cardiothorac Vasc Anesth. 2008;22(3):423–5.
3. Rozner MA. Preoperative evaluations: the very last chance to identify a problem with a pacemaker or implanted cardioverter-defibrillator. J Cardiothorac Vasc Anesth. 2008;22(3):341–6.
4. Suresh M, Benditt DG, Gold B, Joshi GP, Lurie KG. Suppression of cautery-induced electromagnetic interference of cardiac implantable electrical devices by closely spaced bipolar sensing. Anesth Analg. 2011;112(6):1358–61.
5. American Society of Anesthesiologists. Practice advisory for the perioperative management of patients with cardiac implantable electronic devices: pacemakers and implantable cardioverter-defibrillators: an updated report by the American society of anesthesiologists task force on perioperative management of patients with cardiac implantable electronic devices. Anesthesiology. 2011;114(2):247–61.
6. Crossley GH, Poole JE, Rozner MA, Asirvatham SJ, Cheng A, Chung MK, Ferguson TB, Gallagher JD, Gold MR, Hoyt RH, Irefin S, Kusumoto FM, Moorman P, Thompson A. The heart rhythm society expert consensus statement on the perioperative management of patients with implantable defibrillators, pacemakers and arrhythmia monitors: facilities and patient management. j. Published 2011. http://www.hrsonline.org/ClinicalGuidance/cieds_consensus-statement.cfm. Accessed 30 May 2011.
7. Bernstein AD, Daubert JC, Fletcher RD, et al. The revised NASPE/BPEG generic code for antibradycardia, adaptive-rate, and multisite pacing. North American society of pacing and electrophysiology/British pacing and electrophysiology group. Pacing Clin Electrophysiol. 2002;25(2):260–4.
8. Rozner MA. Review of electrical interference in implanted cardiac devices. Pacing Clin Electrophysiol. 2003;26(4 Pt 1):923–5.
9. Lau W, Corcoran SJ, Mond HG. Pacemaker tachycardia in a minute ventilation rate-adaptive pacemaker induced by electrocardiographic monitoring. Pacing Clin Electrophysiol. 2006;29(4):438–40.
10. Standards for basic anesthetic monitoring. American society of anesthesiologists. Published 2005. http://www.asahq.org/publicationsAndServices/standards/02.pdf. Accessed 24 Oct 2009.
11. American Society of Anesthesiologists Task Force on Perioperative Management of Patients with Cardiac Rhythm Management Devices. Practice advisory for the perioperative management of patients with cardiac rhythm management devices: pacemakers and implantable cardioverter-defibrillators: a report by the American society of anesthesiologists task force on perioperative management of patients with cardiac rhythm management devices. Anesthesiology. 2005;103(1):186–98.

12. De Marco M, Maggi S. Evaluation of stray radiofrequency radiation emitted by electrosurgical devices. Phys Med Biol. 2006;51(14):3347–58.

13. Skonieczki BD, Wells C, Wasser EJ, Dupuy DE. Radiofrequency and microwave tumor ablation in patients with implanted cardiac devices: is it safe? Eur J Radiol. 2010;79(3):343–6.

14. Cheng A, Nazarian S, Spragg DD, et al. Effects of surgical and endoscopic electrocautery on modern-day permanent pacemaker and implantable cardioverter-defibrillator systems. Pacing Clin Electrophysiol. 2008;31(3):344–50.

15. Balakrishnan M, Kuriakose R. Endotracheal tube damage during head and neck surgeries as a result of harmonic scalpel® use. Anesthesiology. 2005;102:870–1.

16. Rozner MA. Implantable cardiac pulse generators, pacemakers and cardioverter-defibrillators. In: Miller RD, Eriksson LI, Fleisher LA, editors. Miller's anesthesia. 7th ed. Philadelphia: Churchill Livingstone; 2009.

17. Hammill SC, Kremers MS, Stevenson LW, Heidenreich PA, Lang CM, Curtis JP, Wang Y, Berul CI, Kadish AH, Al-Khatib SM, Pina IL, Walsh MN, Mirro MJ, Lindsay BD, Reynolds MR, Pontzer K, Blum L, Masoudi F, Rumsfeld J, Brindis RG, Review of the registry's fourth year, incorporating lead data and pediatric ICD procedures, and use as a national performance measure. Heart Rhythm 2010;7(9):1340–45.

13. How to Report Adverse Events Related to the Use of Energy Devices in the Operating Room

Charlotte L. Guglielmi

Responding to an adverse incident associated with a medical device must be a team effort. The first and most immediate response must always be to ensure the safety of the patient. Once it is determined that a patient is safe, facilities must have a pathway to respond to the event. Since these events occur infrequently, the practical steps that need to be taken may be forgotten or poorly understood by practitioners. In this chapter, we describe an event response framework for use when devices fail.

Review of the Literature

A search of the literature reveals little on pathways to respond to a device failure. Feigal and associates [1] advocate that the safety and effectiveness of devices can be improved through monitoring of serious low-frequency events. They contend that early identification of problems by health professionals can assist in decreasing device related injuries. Two papers addressed medical device failures attributed to robot-assisted surgery. The first paper, by Dharam et al. used a Web-based survey sent to urologists performing robot-assisted laparoscopic prostatectomy [2]. In addition to demographics and experience, the survey questions included whether the surgeon had experienced a failure, the timing of the failure and the response. The authors concluded that patients should be counseled preoperatively about the risks of failure and surgical teams should have a plan to manage breakdowns. In the second paper, Andonian et al. [3] published a review of the Manufacturer and User Facility Device

L.S. Feldman et al. (eds.), *The SAGES Manual on the Fundamental Use of Surgical Energy (FUSE)*, DOI 10.1007/978-1-4614-2074-3_13, © Springer Science+Business Media, LLC 2012

Experience (MAUDE) database of The United States Food and Drug Administration (FDA) for failures associated with robot-assisted laparoscopic surgeries. Although there is an increase in the number of robotic-assisted surgery related device failures reported to the database, there are few occurrences that result in patient injury [3]. The literature is silent on medical device failures attributed to surgical energy and also does not address a framework that can be utilized to assist surgical teams in managing those failures when they occur.

Mandatory Reporting of Device Failures

The Safe Medical Devices Act of 1990, in accordance with facility policies, requires the monitoring and reporting of incidents in which a medical device is related to the death, serious injury or illness of any individual. Congress enacted this legislation with the goal of increasing the amount of information received about device failures both by the FDA and the manufacturers. As a result of this legislation, the MAUDE database was developed to allow the voluntary reporting of device-related adverse events. The database includes reports entered since 1993 [4].

Twenty-six states have laws in place that require the reporting of adverse events. Twelve of the twenty-six require reporting of the impact of the event on the patient as well as the cause identified in the root cause analysis. The mechanism for reporting varies from state to state [5].

The Joint Commission (TJC) does not stipulate mandatory reporting of device failures in the standards. However, if in the course of a sentinel event review and response a device failure is named as the root cause of an event which resulted in an unanticipated death or major loss of permanent function, the same due diligence and follow-up would be needed. The expectation is that a timely root cause analysis was conducted and an action plan was developed which included identified steps to prevent a reoccurrence of the event, timelines for implementation and steps to evaluate the interventions. Facilities have the ability to define the events as long as they are concurrent with TJC definition of sentinel event [6].

Finally, in 2002, the National Quality Forum (NQF) endorsed a list of serious reportable events (SRE). The goal of the list was to increase public accountability and consumer access to critical information about health-care performance. The SRE list is a consensus document.

Stakeholders from both public and professional sectors as well as accrediting agencies, societies, and industry participated in its development. The list includes 28 SRE which are classified into six categories. One of the categories is product or device events. The second of the three SRE in this category is, "patient death or serious disability associated with the use or function of a device in patient care in which the device is used or functions other than as intended" [7].

Failed Medical Device Response

A medical device is defined as any instrument, apparatus, appliance, material, or health-care product, excluding drugs, used for a patient. A failed device is defined as any device used to provide care to a patient that does not perform according to the manufacturer's specifications that causes injury to, or death of, a patient or that could have caused injury or death without the intervention of a clinician [8]. Examples of devices are an electrosurgical generator (ESU), a dispersive electrode, or the hand-piece from an ultrasonic coagulator.

With regard to energy devices, the generic term *device* can be further broken down to include the instrument (which delivers the energy to the patient), the generator (which creates the energy in the appropriate electrical or mechanical form), the cable (which delivers the energy from the generator to the instrument), and accessories (i.e., dispersive electrodes). Should a device fail to work, misfire, or cause injury to the patient, it should immediately be removed from use. The instrument, cable, generator, and any other items required to deliver care such as the dispersive electrode should be sequestered along with the original packaging. The packaging is needed to determine lot numbers in the event that there is a defect that is broader than the single event that is being reported. It is critical that items not be altered until they have been examined so they should be placed in a biohazardous bag, labeled, and not cleaned or processed. Removing generators from service is critical. Additionally, any error codes that displayed as the device failed should be noted. The meticulous documentation in the operative record of the control numbers of devices is critically important for both the follow-up of a single event or if there is a need to review all cases in which a particular device has been used. Of significant importance is that OR staff be educated not only on how and what to sequester in an event but also on where items should be stored until they are collected for analysis.

Each facility must develop guidelines that clearly outline the immediate steps that occur locally in the operating room as well as the notification chain of command that is to be used to alert designated individuals that a failure has occurred. The extent to which notification occurs is dependent on the severity of the incident. At a minimum, devices failures must be recorded in the facility patient safety reporting system formally known in most hospitals as the incident reporting system. As the process unfolds, Health Care Quality/Risk Management should be consulted at each step of the way.

The guideline should also designate an individual(s) responsible for the follow-up. Role titles for this person vary from facility to facility. Some commonly used titles are Product Safety Coordinator, Clinical Technology Coordinator, or Device Incident Investigator. This person works closely with a designee from Health Care Quality/Risk Management to ensure that all steps of the follow-up and reporting occur to meet regulatory and facility requirements.

As previously noted, any event in which a device failure is suspected should be documented in the facility's patient safety reporting system. This is generally the responsibility of the circulating registered nurse. It ensures documented follow-up to the failure. In the event of injury to a patient, the surgeon should disclose the incident to the patient and complete documentation that is required by the institution. If disclosing an event is difficult for an individual surgeon, specialists from Health Care Quality/Risk Management or surgical leadership should be available to assist in the conversation.

Following the event the Product Safety Coordinator is responsible to document the incident and tie the pieces together. This process should occur regardless if the failure resulted in a patient injury or not. The thrust of the work is to reconstruct the incident. This is accomplished by gathering testimony from the individuals present when the incident occurred, and gathering photographic evidence. Research should be conducted to determine if similar events have occurred at the facility or elsewhere. Frequently, a facility's own as well as the MAUDE and the ECRI Institute's Medical Device Safety Reports (MDSR) databases are consulted. A Clinical Engineer who specializes in the surgical environment should be consulted to conduct a functional test of the

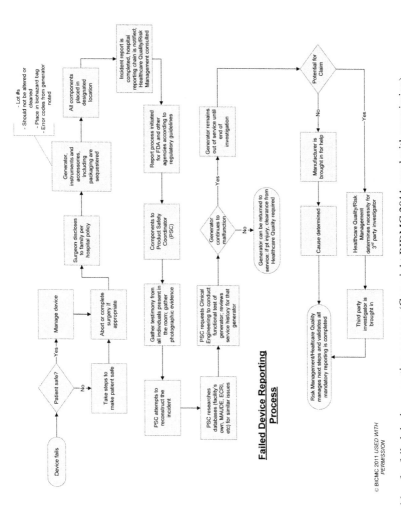

Fig. 13.1. Algorithm for failed device reporting process. (Copyright BIDMC 2011, used with permission).

device and to review the service log for the device. Equipment such as electrosurgical generators should remain out of service until a full inspection has been completed.

In the event that the root cause analysis of the failure is inconclusive, the device manufacturer should be contacted to assist in the investigation. Of note, device manufacturers will consult only on the products that they manufacture. If the components of the system are supplied by multiple vendors an added layer of complexity is introduced as each vendor will address only the product which they manufactured. In cases in which there is potential for a claim, or when the facility and manufacturer have differing perspectives on the causes of the event, Health Care Quality/Risk Management can elect to engage a third party investigator to assist in determining the cause(s). Engagement of a third party investigator rarely occurs except in cases in which a serious injury or patient death has occurred.

The Product Safety Coordinator is also the person who will report the failure to the FDA. The FDA's Medical Product Safety Network (MedSun) is a user-friendly reporting tool that is used by many facilities. Throughout the process, feedback to the point of care staff, surgeons, nurses, and others should be ongoing. A graphic representation of this framework is demonstrated in Fig. 13.1.

The Product Safety Coordinator can also be helpful in sourcing medical devices for known failures. This information should be included in the due diligence that is exercised when a facility is considering new product requests.

Conclusion

A timely and directed response by all members of the surgical team is essential whenever a medical device fails. Beyond meeting the regulatory requirements of reporting, the learning that occurs as a result of the event once disseminated will assist in improving patient outcomes and creating systems that are safer.

Acknowledgment: The author wishes to acknowledge Richard Stroshane, Product Safety Coordinator, Beth Israel Deaconess Medical Center, Boston, MA, for his assistance in the development of this manuscript.

References

1. Feigal D, Gardner S, McClellan M. Ensuring safe and effective medical devices. N Engl J Med. 2003;348(3):191–2.
2. Dharam K, High R, Clark CJ, LaGrange C. Malfunction of the da Vinci robotic system during robot-assisted laparoscopic prostatectomy, an internal survey. J Endourol. 2010;24(4):571–5.
3. Andonian S, Okeke Z, Okeke DA, Rastinehad A, VanderBrink BA, Richstone L, Lee B. Device failures associated with patient injuries during robot-assisted laparoscopic surgeries: a comprehensive review of the FDA MAUDE database. Can J Urol. 2008;15(1):3912–6.
4. How to report a problem (Medical Devices). FDA, U.S. Food and Drug Administration. 2011. http://www.fda.gov/MedicalDevices/Safety/ReportaProblem/default.htm. Accessed on 16 Aug 2011.
5. Adverse events in hospitals: state reporting systems. Department of health and human services, Office of the inspector general, OEI-06-07-00471, Dec 2008. p. 26.
6. Sentinel Events (SE), CAMH refreshed core. The Joint Commission, Jan 2011. SE 1–18.
7. Serious reportable events, NQF (Oct 2008). http://www.qualityforum.org/print_content_details.aspx?title=Serious+Reportable+Events. Accessed 16 Aug 2011.
8. PSM 100-26. Guidelines for compliance with safe medical device act, perioperative services Manual, Beth Israel Deaconess Medical Center, Boston, MA (31 May 2011).

Part II
Enrichment Chapters

14. Hands-On Station: Fundamentals and Safety of Radiofrequency Electrosurgery

Malcolm G. Munro

The objective of this station is for the user to learn to properly set up and use electrosurgery and understand how to achieve desired tissue effects. After completion of this station, the user will be able to set up an electrosurgical unit (generator) with monopolar and bipolar instruments, including selection of appropriate output settings; demonstrate a variety of tissue effects and understand the depth of thermal injury achieved with different generator settings; understand the safety mechanisms in a split-pad dispersive electrode; and demonstrate thermal injury to surrounding tissue with insulated and noninsulated monopolar laparoscopic instruments through a variety of mechanisms (Table 14.1).

Required Materials

- Electrosurgery unit (ESU) with foot pedal
- Dispersive electrodes: One split and one simple
- Flank or skirt steaks—several large pieces
- Hand-activated monopolar device
- Two laparoscopic monopolar instruments and cords, one with damaged insulation
- Uninsulated laparoscopic grasper or other instrument
- Small fluorescent light "bulb" (~15 W)
- Laparoscopic cannulae—metal and plastic, 5–5.5 mm diameter
- Simulated abdominal wall (constructed from rodent screen designed for an external house dryer vent, portions cut out, and flank steak draped as in Fig. 14.1)

This simulation is based on a polymer frame constructed from a rodent screen designed for an external house dryer vent (Fig. 14.1).

L.S. Feldman et al. (eds.), *The SAGES Manual on the Fundamental Use of Surgical Energy (FUSE)*, DOI 10.1007/978-1-4614-2074-3_14,
© Springer Science+Business Media, LLC 2012

Table 14.1. Laboratory station fundamentals and safety.

	Component	Equipment	Exercise
ESU basics	Generator demonstration	ESU, foot pedal, monopolar cord for monopolar laparoscopic instruments, generic bipolar cable for bipolar instruments, matching bipolar laparoscopic instrument, dispersive electrodes, fruit or tissue	Demonstrate ESU components, jacks, displays, controls, in the context of a circuit with a bipolar instrument, and a monopolar instrument and dispersive electrode
Tissue effects	Vaporization/Cutting	ESU, monopolar hand instrument-electrode with blade electrode, dispersive electrode, tissue, scalpel	Demonstrate vaporization and linear extension using edge of blade electrode at low voltage; similar to using blended and high voltage ("coag") outputs. Scalpel to cut tissue to demonstrate gross thermal damage
	Coagulation/Desiccation	Same as above	Use same outputs and settings with same electrode turned to side to lower power density
	Fulguration	Same as above	Demonstrate fulguration using same output wattage but high voltage waveform

Dispersive electrode	Split electrode	ESU, flank or skirt steak	Activate ESU while peeling back tissue demonstrating alarm
	Standard (not split) electrode	ESU, flank or skirt steak	Activate ESU while peeling back tissue demonstrating that alarm will not activate—try to demonstrate capacity for tissue injury when power density is high
Current diversion	Insulation break	Laparoscopic monopolar hand instrument with pinhole defect	Demonstrate capacity of the laparoscopic hand instrument to create tissue damage
	Direct	Noninsulated laparoscopic instrument and insulated monopolar laparoscopic hand instrument	Demonstrate remote tissue damage using direct coupling from an activated monopolar instrument's electrode to a conductive hand instrument (e.g., probe, driver)
	Capacitative	8–15 W Fluorescent light, ESU, monopolar instrument, dispersive electrode	Use light to show difference between voltage of the two main outputs, show capacitative capability in open circuit

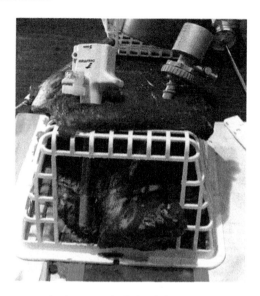

Fig. 14.1. Laparoscopic electrosurgical simulation setup.

Portions of the grid composition are cut out. Two pieces of flank steak are sutured together and the steak is placed on the dispersive electrode which is, in turn, attached to the ESU. Then the frame is placed on the steak while the rest of the meat is wrapped around the back to the top of the frame in a manner that simulates the abdominal wall. Laparoscopic cannulas are added. Tissue can be placed in the peritoneal cavity (on the steak "floor") to act as a target for the electrosurgical demonstrations. The frame can be easily cleaned for resuse.

Electrosurgical Units (Generators)

This is the introductory component of this station where the instructor reviews the basic design and function of an electrosurgical generator (Fig. 14.2). Teaching points include the following:

1. The connection to simple 50 Hz 110 V alternating current (AC) from a standard wall outlet.
2. The jack for the dispersive electrode includes demonstration of the differences between the impedance monitored electrode (generally a "split pad") and simple dispersive electrodes without impedance monitoring.

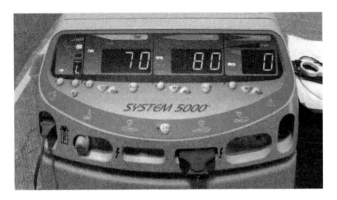

Fig. 14.2. Basic design and function of an electrosurgical generator.

3. The jacks for the unipolar instruments/cords and the bipolar instruments/cords. Included in this demonstration is the nature of the cord/cables for the two different systems. Bipolar cables have at least two wires reflecting the fact that both electrodes are in the instrument, while cables for unipolar systems typically have a single wire, reflecting that the instrument has only one electrode.

4. Understanding the LED panels that display the settings of the high voltage, low voltage, and, if so equipped, the bipolar outputs (low voltage).

5. If they are present, know the differences between the "subsettings" for the high voltage (e.g., "spray," "fulgurate") and the low voltage (e.g., "pure," "blend") outputs.

6. Know where the footpedal jack is and how it impacts the use of devices.

Demonstration of Tissue Effects

A piece of flank or skirt steak is placed on a dispersive electrode with appropriate settings on the generator—e.g., 50 W low voltage, "pure" ("cut") and 50 W, high voltage "spray" ("coag"). A simple hand-activated blade electrode is the best example and fits with the demonstration in the presentation and text of the chapter.

1. Vaporization/cutting: Use the low voltage output to demonstrate the use of the edge of a blade electrode to focally and linearly vaporize (cut) tissue. Create three parallel (about

1 cm apart) 1 cm deep incisions with the "pure cut," a "blend" output as well as the high voltage "coag" output. The trainee notes the ease of cutting, the appearance of visible sparking, and the gross thermal injury below the incision line. Then using a simple scalpel, an incision is made perpendicular to the direction of the incisions so that a gross comparison of thermal depth of injury can be made.

2. Desiccation/coagulation: Using the same blade electrode, at the same "pure cut" output settings (e.g., 50 W), the tissue is touched with the wide side of the blade and the ESU is activated. The trainees should appreciate the absence of vaporization and the presence of tissue coagulation. The scalpel can be used to expose the deeper tissues.

3. Fulguration: The same blade electrode can be used (should be as clean as possible) but the "blue" hand button or the "coag" footpedal should be depressed to activate the high voltage output. The electrode is held about 1–3 mm from the tissue, and the arcing is demonstrated as fulguration is performed without touching the electrode to the tissue. If the generator is so equipped, there can be a demonstration of the differences between the "fulgurate" and "spray" modes. The trainee should observe the carbonization associated with the coagulated and desiccated tissue. The scalpel can be used to create an incision demonstrating the superficial nature of the thermal injury.

Dispersive Electrode and Safety Mechanisms

The demonstration is performed with an ESU, a piece of skirt or flank steak about 12×20 cm, two dispersive electrodes, one "split" and the other not split, and a simple blade electrode with a hand toggle or other type of switch (Fig. 14.3).

1. The "split" dispersive electrode is plugged into the ESU. The trainee notes that the alarm lights up on the ESU panel reflecting the fact that there is no tissue in contact with the electrode. Attempts to activate the "active" electrode for tissue cutting or hemostasis fail.

2. The steak is placed over the dispersive electrode covering the two sides of the pad. The trainee should note that the lighted alarm signal on the ESU goes out, and one can activate the active electrode.

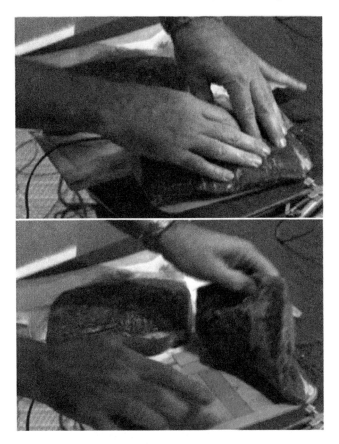

Fig. 14.3. The demonstration of dispersive electrode and safety mechanisms is performed with an ESU, a piece of skirt or flank steak about 12×20 cm, two dispersive electrodes, one "split" and the other not split, and a simple blade electrode with a hand toggle or other type of switch.

3.   The steak surrogate is partially peeled from the "tissue" until the dispersive electrode alarm illuminates. This will occur typically if about $30\% \pm$ of the entire electrode is detached. Attempts to activate the active electrode will fail.

4.   The split electrode is removed from the ESU while leaving the power on.

5.   The simple dispersive electrode is then plugged in, and the trainee will note that the ESU alarm does not go on (compare with the split dispersive electrode where the alarm would activate).

6. The steak is removed from the split dispersive electrode and placed on the simple dispersive electrode.
7. The instructor can carefully peel back the steak from the dispersive electrode while the system is activated until the current density (amount of tissue in contact with the dispersive electrode) is high enough that sparking or tissue trauma is seen to occur.

Current Diversion

This demonstration is performed with a number of tools that include the ESU, a laparoscopic monopolar instrument, a simple or split dispersive electrode, a monopolar cord, and a small fluorescent light "bulb" of about 15 W. A surrogate for the abdominal wall and peritoneal cavity can be created with a modified rodent vent grid and a large piece of skirt or flank steak (Fig. 14.4). Laparoscopic cannulas are needed and it is useful to have both metal and plastic versions, preferably with 5–5.5 mm internal diameter. If it is difficult to get a large area piece of skirt or flank steak, two pieces can be sutured together with three to four interrupted box sutures.

1. *Insulation break*: For this demonstration, a disposable monopo-lar laparoscopic hand instrument is carefully damaged by

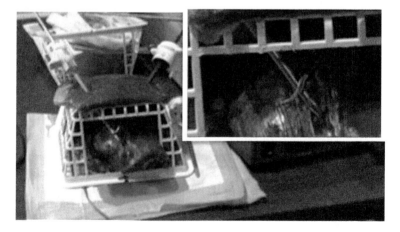

Fig. 14.4. For this current diversion exercise, an intact monopolar laparoscopic hand instrument is placed through one access port, while another uninsulated hand instrument is passed through another port.

making a pinhole in the insulation. The instrument is then attached to the generator and passed through the laparoscopic access port. The instrument is activated, first with low voltage, then with high voltage output with the pinhole-damaged portion in close proximity to surrogate tissue. The trainee should be able to see the local arcing and damage created on the underlying tissue.

2. *Direct coupling*: An intact monopolar laparoscopic hand instrument is placed through one access port, while another uninsulated hand instrument is passed through another port. The unipolar instrument is activated while touching the non-insulated device, which, in turn is near to target tissue (a portion of flank steak placed appropriately on the tissue substrate that lays on the dispersive electrode (Fig. 14.4)).

3. *Capacitative coupling*: First the energy around the activated but insulated and intact laparoscopic monopolar hand instrument is demonstrated using the light bulb in the context of an open circuit. Settings for this exercise vary with the generators but should be identical on the low ("cut") and high ("coag") outputs to demonstrate the voltage differences between the two. Typically settings between 50 and 70 W work, and it is preferable to use the "spray" setting on the "coag" output if it is available.

   (a) Capacitative charge: A monopolar laparoscopic or hand instrument is attached to the generator. The dispersive electrode should be attached so that the alarm is off using either a simple, single pad, or a split pad with a quarter of tissue bridging the gap between the two pad electrodes. The bulb is held near to the laparoscopic hand electrode or the cord of either of the electrodes and the generator is activated. In some instances, if there is difficulty with illumination, the cord can be wrapped around the bulb (Fig. 14.5). The instructor should be able to demonstrate the differences in voltage by the distance between the wire/electrode required to light the bulb. The distance required for illumination using the high voltage "coag" output should be less than that for the low voltage "cut" output.

   (b) Capacitative coupling and tissue injury.

      i. For this exercise, set up based on number 3a (above), the capacitative charge in an open circuit is used to demonstrate the potential for inadvertent tissue injury. The instructor wraps the monopolar cord around his neck. The shaft of a monopolar laparoscopic hand

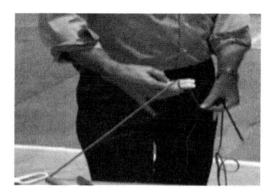

Fig. 14.5. For this capacitative coupling and tissue injury exercise, the capacitative charge in an open circuit is used to demonstrate the potential for inadvertent tissue injury.

instrument is held in one hand near to the tissue on the dispersive electrode but is not attached to the cord. The ESU is activated and the trainees are asked to note the arcing of current and the resulting tissue effect that should be recognized with each output (low voltage and high voltage) but may be more recognizable with the high voltage because of the arcing.

ii. For this exercise, two monopolar laparoscopic hand instruments, two plastic 5 mm cannulas, the ESU with a foot pedal, and the abdominal wall/laparoscopic model are required. One of the hand electrodes is attached to the generator and high voltage output, approximately 80 W is set. Both instruments are passed into the surrogate peritoneal cavity via the positioned cannulas. The attached electrode is used to fulgurate or cause other tissue effects on the target tissue. Then the active electrode in the attached instrument is lifted off the tissue 1+ cm, and the "free" instrument is brought near the target as the ESU is activated. The trainees should see a tissue effect generated near the free instrument's tip secondary to capacitative coupling through the individual holding the instruments.

15. Hands-on Station: Art and Science of Monopolar Electrosurgery – Case Studies of Metal-to-Metal Arcing and Single Port Cannula Surgery

C. Randle Voyles

Enhanced "artful" application of monopolar electrosurgery occurs only after a period of continued real-time study in animate in vivo models. The models outlined in the previous chapter (Chap. 14) with steak on a dispersive electrode are useful for outlining concepts and poorly understood principles. For example, the novice surgeon can demonstrate the various tissue effects of concentration of current at various wattages. Further demonstrations outlined how current can be inadvertently concentrated at unintended sites through direct coupling, insulation failure, or induced/capacitive coupling. Enhanced art forms occur as a function of insightful study. In this station, issues surrounding the risks of application of electrosurgery to staple lines and with single port laparoscopic surgery will be demonstrated.

Required Material and Equipment

- Electrosurgical unit (generator).
- Dispersive electrode.
- Flank steaks.
- Staples—straightened out.
- Laparoscopic monopolar instrument.
- Laparoscopic monopolar instrument with defective insulation.
- Laparoscopic grasper.
- Multichannel single port trocar.
- Laparoscope.
- Laparoscopic setup as in Chap. 14.

L.S. Feldman et al. (eds.), *The SAGES Manual on the Fundamental Use of Surgical Energy (FUSE)*, DOI 10.1007/978-1-4614-2074-3_15,
© Springer Science+Business Media, LLC 2012

Two further demonstrations are useful to outline understanding of concepts.

Demonstration 1: Direct Coupling to Staple Line Generates 1,000°C

To outline the maximum effect of concentrated current, a staple (from either a paper stapler or preferably from one of the mechanical stapling devices) is straightened and one half of the length is inserted into the steak on the dispersive electrode as in the previously outlined model. The surgical electrode is activated (open circuit) and held near enough to the staple to allow continuous arcing with "coag" mode at 40–60 W power. In short order, the staple will melt and disintegrate. Do you understand the biophysics of this demonstration? Do you "see" maximum current density with maximum thermal change that can be generated in a laparoscopic setting with monopolar electrosurgery?

A more telling model of the same demonstration can be accomplished in the operating room. After the end of colon resection, take the resected colon and place it on a dispersive electrode. Arrange the colon so that the surgical electrode approximates the "end staple" of the transected bowel (Fig. 15.1a); activate the electrode so that there is a continuous arc to the staple (Fig. 15.1b); be careful to observe the disintegration of the staple with an explosion of "staple shrapnel" (Fig. 15.1c) as the high levels of heat cause instant boiling of the tissue in association with the staple line (Fig. 15.1d).

Now reflect back on a capillary ooze at a stapled anastomosis. Be careful using energy on the staple line (or near clips) as the same demonstration can be affected with a resultant anastomotic failure in 3–5 days.

Demonstration 2: Amplified Electrosurgical Risk of Stray Current with Single Port Surgery

Use the same model outlined in the previous chapter (simulation of the abdominal cavity), but use a multichannel single port trocar to introduce the closely aligned instruments. Do several tasks:

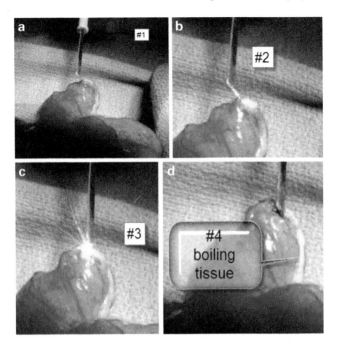

Fig. 15.1. (**a**) The colon is arranged so that the surgical electrode approximates the "end staple" of the transected bowel. (**b**) The electrode is activated so that there is a continuous arc to the staple. (**c**) The staple will disintegrate with an explosion of "staple shrapnel." (**d**) The high levels of heat cause instant boiling of the tissue in association with the staple line.

1. Introduce a surgical electrode alongside a laparoscope. Demonstrate how readily the active electrode can contact the laparoscope and deliver energy to an unintended site (Notice how the instruments are in closer proximity to one another than with conventional port technology).

2. Introduce the instrument with known defective insulation. Is it apparent that the chance for injury has been enhanced by single port introduction?

3. Activate the electrode open circuit (not touching tissue) and advance another inactive electrode through alongside the active electrode. Advance the "inactive electrode" to near the steak and observe the stray "induced" current onto the "inactive" electrode. Change the ESU output from 20 to 100 W "coag" and observe the qualitative differences in induced currents. Now do the same with "cut" current (low voltage) with very little induced current.

16. Hands-on Station: Thermal Spread with Bipolar Electrosurgery

Dean Mikami

The purpose of this station is for the user to demonstrate the safe use of bipolar devices in the laparoscopic setting. After completion of this station, the user will be able to set up and demonstrate the safe use of a laparoscopic bipolar instrument while completing a simple surgical task. The user will transect ex vivo tissue while recognizing and controlling thermal spread. The equipment needed for the lab is listed below. A thermal imaging camera can be used to monitor the user's thermal spread during the task (Fig. 16.1).

Required Material and Equipment

- Flank steak: 4×4×0.5 in.
- One or more bipolar instrument of choice.
- Laparoscopic trainer box (e.g., SAGES FLS Trainer Box™).
- Thermal imaging camera.
- Infrared thermometer.
- Preconstructed surgical pathway (Fig. 16.2).

A preconstructed surgical pathway of corkboard and metal wire is used (Fig. 16.2) to create a path for the surgeon through which to navigate a bipolar surgical instrument, while keeping the thermal spread within the wired boundary. In order for the user to have a realistic experience in the ex vivo setup, a 4×4×0.5 in. flank steak is used as the tissue model (Fig. 16.3). The task is performed within a laparoscopic training box, such as the FLS™ box available through SAGES (Fig. 16.4).

L.S. Feldman et al. (eds.), *The SAGES Manual on the Fundamental Use of Surgical Energy (FUSE)*, DOI 10.1007/978-1-4614-2074-3_16, © Springer Science+Business Media, LLC 2012

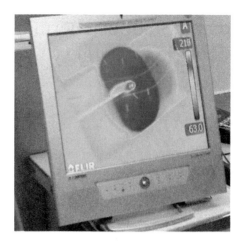

Fig. 16.1. Thermal spread from bipolar instrument demonstrated with thermal imaging camera.

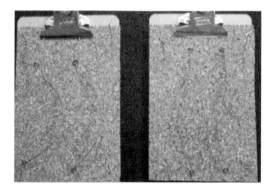

Fig. 16.2. Preconstructed surgical pathway and grid.

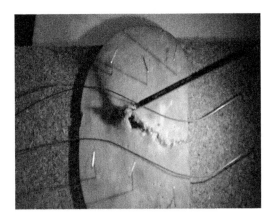

Fig. 16.3. Flank steak model with wire path boundary.

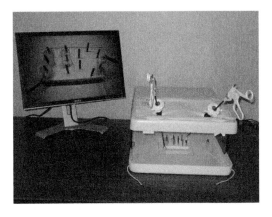

Fig. 16.4. SAGES FLS trainer box™. (Image used with permission of SAGES).

17. Hands-on Station: Ultrasonic Energy Devices

Dana D. Portenier

Required Materials

- Ultrasonic shears and generators (various vendors).
- Flank steak.
- Bovine liver/gallbladder tissue block (optional).
- Temperature gun infrared thermometer (can be purchased at most hardware stores for approximately $40).
- Laparoscopic trainer box (optional).

Instrument Setup

This is the introductory component of this station where the instructor reviews the basic design and function of the devices. The instructor should:

1. Demonstrate correct set up of the generator, connection of the device, and initial testing of the instrument based upon manufacture recommendations.
2. Review the error codes that may display upon the generator.
3. Demonstrate the proper use of the device settings. Discuss the differences in effects and clinical indications for use of each setting.

L.S. Feldman et al. (eds.), *The SAGES Manual on the Fundamental Use of Surgical Energy (FUSE)*, DOI 10.1007/978-1-4614-2074-3_17, © Springer Science+Business Media, LLC 2012

Instrument Use

The instructor reviews the use of the device. This may be done in a laparoscopic trainer box. The instructor should:

1. Demonstrate proper use of the device on either liver/gallbladder tissue block or flank steak.
2. Demonstrate heat generated during tissue activation using temperature gun infrared thermometer.
3. Demonstrate techniques to rapidly cool the blade prior to dissection on critical structures, including touching noncritical tissue. Use the thermometer to show the cooling effect.

18. Hands-on Station: Cavitron Ultrasonic Surgical Aspirator (CUSA) and Argon Beam Device

James S. Choi

Required Materials

- CUSA system and handpieces.
- Argon beam system with handpieces and/or foot pedal.
- Target tissue: bovine liver.

CUSA Demonstration

1. The bovine liver tissue is placed on a table.
2. The CUSA device is set up as shown according to manufacturer's recommendations.
3. The liver capsule is cut with a scalpel.
4. The CUSA system is used to dissect through the liver tissue. The CUSA handpiece is held like a pencil, without squeezing the flue (Fig. 18.1). With the other hand, gentle traction and countertraction is applied to the target liver tissue, and the CUSA handpiece is applied in a very gentle manner over the liver tissue to be fragmented and aspirated. The liver tissue is aspirated away, leaving blood vessels and bile ducts behind.

L.S. Feldman et al. (eds.), *The SAGES Manual on the Fundamental
Use of Surgical Energy (FUSE)*, DOI 10.1007/978-1-4614-2074-3_18,
© Springer Science+Business Media, LLC 2012

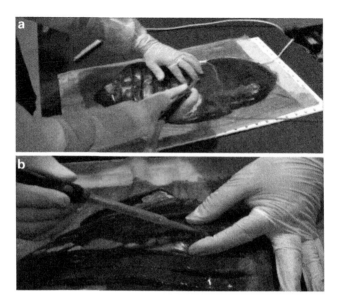

Fig. 18.1. (**a**) The CUSA handpiece is held like a pencil. (**b**) After the liver capsule is incised, the CUSA device is used to dissect through the liver tissue. The liver tissue is aspirated by the device, leaving blood vessels and bile ducts behind.

Argon Beam Device Demonstration

1. The bovine liver tissue is placed on a table.
2. The Argon beam system is set up as shown according to manufacturer's recommendations.
3. The argon beam handpiece is held like a pencil, and the tip is placed over the liver tissue without making contact with the target tissue. The handpiece is activated by the button on the handpiece or the foot pedal. A small stream of argon beam will emanate from the handpiece tip to the target liver tissue. The tip of the handpiece should not come in direct contact with the target tissue.

19. Hands-on Station: Radiofrequency Ablation

Pascal R. Fuchshuber

The objective of this station is for the user to demonstrate the use of RFA on bovine liver. After completion of this station, the user will be able to set up an RFA device; demonstrate heat transfer from the ablation zone; demonstrate proper placement of the active electrode in a target lesion under ultrasound guidance; and demonstrate the effect of a heat sink. The equipment needed for the lab set up is listed below.

Required Material and Equipment

- One or more RFA systems of choice.
- One or more US systems of choice.
- Target tissue: bovine liver.
- Target: small olive without pit.
- Several dispersive electrodes.
- Several active electrodes.
- Flexible copper wire.
- Surgical knife.
- Mayo Clamp.
- Gloves.

Setup

A dispersive electrode is placed face up onto the table, and a portion of a bovine liver (minimally mois) is carefully laid on the dispersive electrode. The electrosurgical RFA unit is connected to a standard electrical outlet and activated. The active electrode is connected to the unit.

L.S. Feldman et al. (eds.), *The SAGES Manual on the Fundamental Use of Surgical Energy (FUSE)*, DOI 10.1007/978-1-4614-2074-3_19,
© Springer Science+Business Media, LLC 2012

An intraoperative ultrasound (US) unit is turned on and placed at one end of the table with a small intraoperative ultrasound probe attached (Figs. 19.1 and 19.2). It is important to dry the liver pieces before placing them on the dispersive electrode to prevent too much fluid accumulation. This can be easily done by blotting with dry paper towels. Frequently change the liver tissue as previous ablation zones will interfere with new simulations.

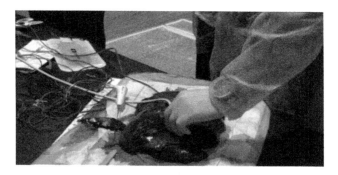

Fig. 19.1. Table setup for RFA simulation. Large piece of bovine liver is placed over a dispersive electrode (*blue* connection cable). Ultrasound of the liver is performed. Active electrode is seen to the *left* of the liver.

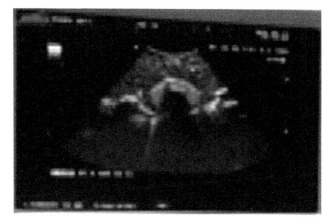

Fig. 19.2. Ultrasound setup showing a picture of a target lesion (olive) within the liver parenchyma (*round shadow*).

Demonstrations

1. *Passive burn of adjacent tissue.* This simulation is designed to show the potential for thermal injury of an adjacent organ due to heat transfer from the ablation zone. Two separate pieces of liver are used. An active electrode is placed into one of the two pieces near the surface ("active tissue"). A second piece ("passive tissue") is placed so it touches the first piece in the vicinity of the active electrode. Perform an RFA cycle for 5 min at 100° target temperature. Observe the "blanching" of the passive tissue due to thermal conduction from the hot surface of the "active" tissue.

2. *Proper placement of active electrode.* This simulation is designed to teach the proper placement of the active electrode with regard to the target lesion. Make a small cut on a piece of liver and force a small olive as deep into the liver tissue as possible. The user should explain the proper function and settings and then activate the electrosurgical RFA unit. The active electrode is then placed under US guidance correctly into the target and a complete ablation cycle for the size of the target is performed. The liver tissue is cut after completion to demonstrate an ablation zone that should completely encompass the target. Discuss if that has not occurred and why (Figs. 19.3 and 19.4).

3. *Simulation of heat/electrical sink.* This simulation is designed to show the heat/electrical sink produced by a large blood vessel

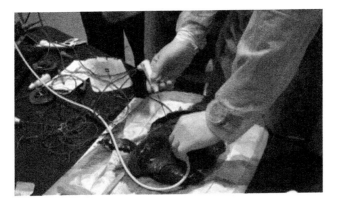

Fig. 19.3. Activating the electrosurgical RFA unit and explaining the function and settings.

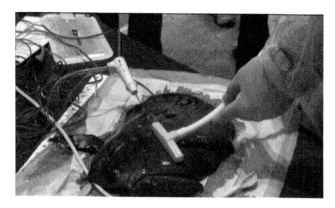

Fig. 19.4. Placement of the active electrode under US guidance into the liver tissue.

in the vicinity of the ablation. Place a small olive as a target into a piece of liver. Splice the copper wire to the dispersive electrode wire and introduce the copper wire with the help of a Mayo Clamp into the liver tissue in proximity to the target/olive (2–3 cm). After completing an ablation, cut the liver to show the target and wire. Observe the thermal destruction of tissue surrounding the copper wire as simulation of diversion of electrical/energy away from the target lesion by a large blood vessel.

20. Hands-on Station: Microwave Devices

Ryan Z. Swan and David A. Iannitti

Experiment Number 1: Ex Vivo Microwave Ablation Model

Equipment

1. Microwave ablation (MWA) system.
    (a) Microwave generator.
    (b) Microwave antenna.
        i. Saline perfusion tubing and 1-L bags of normal saline for internally cooled transcutaneous MWA antennas.
2. Tissue.
    (a) Porcine or bovine kidney and liver.
    (b) Water bath to warm tissue to 37°C prior to ablation.
    (c) Scalpel and metric ruler to transect and measure tissue.

Experimental Setup

1. Compare ablation volume after MWA at different power and time settings within one tissue type. This experiment will give the user an idea of how these settings can be manipulated to effect ablation size; however, these experimental dimensions may not represent true ablation zone dimensions in perfused human tissue during actual clinical ablation.
    (a) Variable time settings.
        i. 2–6 min.

L.S. Feldman et al. (eds.), *The SAGES Manual on the Fundamental Use of Surgical Energy (FUSE)*, DOI 10.1007/978-1-4614-2074-3_20,
© Springer Science+Business Media, LLC 2012

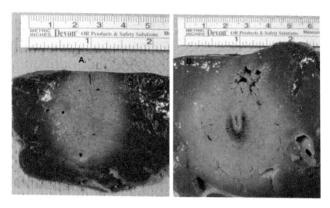

Fig. 20.1. Cross-sections of bovine liver following MWA with a 1.8mm antenna for 4 minutes at 60 W (**a**) and 120 W (**b**).

(b) Variable power settings.
  i. Manufacturer recommended minimum to maximum settings.
(c) Following ablation, allow tissue to cool for 10 min and section the tissue along the axis of the antenna in two perpendicular planes. The zone of ablation is readily identified and can be measured (Fig. 20.1). The volume of ablation can be calculated.
  i. Ablation volume $(cm^3) = [4/3\pi\,(x/2)(y/2)(z/2)]$, where x is the long axis along the ablation antenna and y and z are the short axes perpendicular to the antenna and to each other.
2. Compare ablation volume after MWA at the same time and power settings in different tissue types (Fig. 20.2). This experiment demonstrates the effect of different tissue types with different permittivity (see Chap. 10) on ablation volume.
  (a) Ablation settings: Choose one power and time setting for all ablations.
  (b) Tissue type: Compare bovine or porcine muscle, kidney, and liver ablation dimensions and volume by transecting tissue as above.

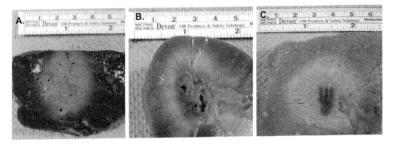

Fig. 20.2. Cross-sections of bovine liver (**a**), porcine kidney (**b**), and porcine muscle (**c**) following MWA with a 1.8-mm antenna for 4 min at 60 W.

Experiment 2: Ex Vivo Demonstration of Microwave Ablation Body Wall Burns

Equipment

1. Microwave ablation system as in experiment 1.
    (a) The user should employ both a surgical MWA antenna and a transcutaneous MWA that are equipped with an internal cooling system.
2. Tissue.
    (a) Bovine liver.
    (b) Bovine or porcine skeletal muscle thinly cut (approximately 2–3 cm thick) to approximate abdominal wall musculature.
    (c) Water bath to warm tissue to 37°C prior to ablation.
    (d) Scalpel and metric ruler to transect and measure tissue.
    (e) Standard laboratory hardware set.
        i. Two support stands with vertical rods and two adjustable clamp attachments on each rod.

Experimental Setup

1. Create an air gap between the target MWA tissue and the substitute body wall and perform MWA by inserting the MW antenna through the body wall (skeletal muscle) into the target tissue (bovine liver). This experiment will demonstrate to the user the complication of abdominal wall burns with improper insertion of the MWA antenna. This experiment also demonstrates the need to create and maintain adequate distance between the target ablation tissue and adjacent structures, as microwave energy will heat tissue across an air gap (see Chap. 10).

   (a) Secure the skeletal muscle to the support scaffolding by clamping each end and suspend it 2–3 cm above the ablation target (bovine liver) to maintain an air gap.

   (b) Insert the MW ablation antenna through the skeletal muscle into the bovine liver and perform a MW ablation.

      i. Choose a high power setting and longer duration for demonstration purposes.

      ii. Ablation effect (tissue cooking and boiling) can be observed in the skeletal muscle around the antenna.

   (c) Following MWA, remove and transect the skeletal muscle to demonstrate the burn, which can be full thickness.

   (d) If available, repeat the MW ablation with two or more antennas in an "array." Some MWA systems allow for more than one generator and antenna to be deployed simultaneously in this fashion.

      i. Vary the spacing between the antennas and vary the angles of insertion. Spacing less than 1.5 cm apart and/or placing the antennas in a nonparallel (converging or diverging) fashion will allow for reflected MW energy to propagate up the antenna shafts and can cause abdominal wall damage (Fig. 20.3).

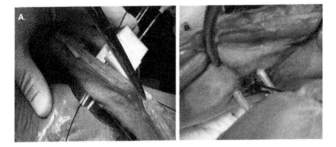

Fig. 20.3. (**a, b**) Experimental model performed in our laboratory utilizing full thickness porcine abdominal wall in a postmortem animal model and bovine liver as the target tissue to examine MWA-induced skin burns when using a three antenna array with variable spacing and angle of insertion.

(e) If available, repeat the above experimental design comparing surgical and transcutaneous antenna designs with one MWA system. Transcutaneous MW ablation systems come equipped with an internal cooling system to control antenna shaft temperatures and prevent body wall burns while antennas intended for surgical use do not.

21. Hands-on Station: Effects of Monopolar and Bipolar Electrosurgery on Cardiovascular Implantable Electrical (Pacemakers or Implanted Cardioverter Defibrillator) Devices

Marc A. Rozner and Stephanie B. Jones

Objectives of This Workstation

1. Understanding of the interaction(s)—primarily the creation of electromagnetic interference (EMI)—between electrosurgical (ES) instruments and cardiovascular implantable (pacemaker [PM] or implanted cardioverter defibrillator (ICD)) devices (CIED).

2. Demonstrate how the presumed current path from the hand tool to the dispersal pad (for ES with a monopolar instrument) can influence the creation of electromagnetic interference.

3. For any given ES presumed current path and instrument:

   (a) Evaluate the effects of electrosurgical unit (generator) power level and settings (coag vs. blend vs. cut) on the creation of EMI during tissue coagulation or cutting.

   (b) Examine the effects of applying the monopolar ES hand tool to an instrument (i.e., tissue equivalent), rather than directly to tissue.

   (c) Examine the effects of allowing the ES hand tool tip to create electrical sparking, rather than a continuous application to the tissue. Note that sparking can also occur when applying the hand tool to a skin edge.

L.S. Feldman et al. (eds.), *The SAGES Manual on the Fundamental Use of Surgical Energy (FUSE)*, DOI 10.1007/978-1-4614-2074-3_21, © Springer Science+Business Media, LLC 2012

(d) Evaluate the extent of EMI from activation of the monopolar ES hand tool at various power levels without touching any tissue or tissue equivalent.
(e) Evaluate the extent to which EMI will occur in lengthy application of ES energy vs. short bursts.

Equipment Needed

- Standard multi-lead electrocardiographic display.
- Patient heart simulator (PHS)—for this demonstration, a unique device was created that allowed control of the "patient's underlying heart rhythm" and electrocardiographic P–R interval. The PHS had ports for connection to a conventional pacemaker or ICD header ports using IS-1 bipolar header connectors. The PHS had an output for an ECG monitor display, and it created ECG pacing artifacts, ECG P waves, and ECG QRS–T complexes that could be displayed on the ECG monitor. If the PHS created the QRS, then the ECG would display a narrow complex and normal appearing QRS–T waveform, but if the CIED created the QRS then the QRS–T waveform would be drawn as a left-bundle branch configuration.
- Conventional pacemaker or ICD generator.
- Manufacturer-specific programmer for the generator listed above to interrogate the CIED and reprogram it.
- Electrosurgical unit capable of using both monopolar and bipolar tools, along with appropriate hand tools and dispersal pads.
- Several metal basins (bread pans).
- Several plastic basins (emesis basins).
- Towels.
- Insulated copper wire.
- Normal saline, water, and conductive gel.
- Alligator clip jumper cables—46 cm × 22 or 24 gauge.
- The "dispersal pad site" was simulated using two identical metal basins to accommodate a split-foil type of dispersal pad. The dispersal pad was cut to separate the two foil sides, and each foil was attached to a basin. Saline was added to each basin, and towels (green surgical) were cut to line and insulate the basins. Insulation was removed from about 6 cm on each

end of a 12-gauge solid copper wire, and the ends were placed into the basins, using the towels and care to ensure that no part of the uninsulated copper was allowed to touch the metal of the bans. The basins were not permitted to contact each other. The split foil pad was connected to the ES generator, and water or ultrasonic gel was mixed with the saline until ES generator reported appropriate "skin integrity."

- The "thorax" was created using a plastic basin filled with saline. Into this basin the "cardiac ends" of both a bipolar atrial pacing lead and a bipolar ventricular pacing lead were placed. These ends were connected using alligator clip wires to the appropriate PHS atrial and ventricular connectors. Pieces of green towel were placed into the bath to cover the atrial and ventricular electrode ends to keep them from making contact with each other. The IS-1 header pins from these leads were inserted into appropriate ports on a CIED generator, and the CIED programmer was used to determine atrial and ventricular lead impedance. If the lead impedances were less than 300 ohms, then conductive gel and water were mixed with the saline to reduce the sodium concentration of the fluid until the pacing impedances were greater than 300 Ω to keep from tripping the "low impedance lead alert" in the CIED.

- For the experiments, the CIED generator was set to DDD mode, 75 bpm, AVd (both pace and sense) 180 ms, atrial fibrillation detect rate 170 bpm, atrial fibrillation pacing VVI mode switch pacing rate 100 bpm)[1]. Atrial sensitivity was 1 mV, ventricular sensitivity was 2 mV, and all pacing outputs were 2 V/0.5 ms. These settings are typical in patients, and more than a 2:1 margin existed for both "sensing" and "pacing" with testing prior to experimental use. To avoid confusion, the "noise reversion pacing" feature (programmable in this CIED) was disabled.

- The ES "surgical site" was prepared in a plastic basin, and it consisted of a balled-up piece of green towel in saline.

---

[1] High-frequency EMI (noise) on the atrial lead is usually interpreted as "atrial fibrillation" by most CIEDs enter "mode switch," at which time the CIED (1) will no longer track atrial depolarizations into the ventricle and (2) creates a mode switch log entry. By setting the mode switch pacing rate to 100 bpm, entry into mode switch becomes easily recognizable (without mode switch the pacing rate will be 75 bpm, unless EMI is entering on the ventricular channel, at which time the pacing rate will fall to 40 bpm).

- The patient simulator was set to 40 bpm with P–R interval 350 ms. On this PHS, the output amplitudes, output pulse widths, and lead sensitivities were not programmable.

The experimental setup consisted of two configurations:

Model 1

The presumed current path went from the "surgical site" through the "thorax" to the "dispersal pad site," which would represent a typical head and neck case with the dispersal pad on a thigh or buttock (this is not the ideal configuration for patient care). To create this model, insulation was removed from about 6 cm on each end of a 12-gauge solid copper wire, one end was placed into one of the "dispersal pad site" basins and the other end was placed into the "thorax" basin. Care was taken to ensure that no part of any uninsulated copper was allowed to touch any metal of the basin, any other uninsulated copper wire, the conductive ends of the pacing electrodes, or the alligator leads. Another similarly prepared copper wire went from the "thorax" basin to the "surgical site" basin. Similar precautions were taken with respect to other metal conductive surfaces. The intent was to use the liquid in the basins as the conductors (Fig. 21.1).

Model 2

The presumed current path went from the "surgical site" to the "dispersal pad site" without crossing the chest, intending to shield the "thorax" from the ES current. This model simulates a typical pelvic case with the dispersal pad on the thigh or buttock, or a head and neck case with the dispersal pad on the posterior-superior shoulder contralateral to the CIED generator. To create this model, insulation was removed from about 6 cm on each end of a 12-gauge solid copper wire, one end was placed into the "dispersal pad site" basin and the other end was placed into the "thorax" basin. Care was taken to ensure that no part of any uninsulated copper was allowed to touch any metal pan or any other uninsulated copper or the conductive ends of the pacing electrodes or alligator leads. Another similarly prepared copper wire went from one of the "dispersal pad site" basins to the "surgical site" basin. Similar precautions were taken with respect to other metal conductive surfaces. The intent was to use the liquid in the basins as the conductors (Fig. 21.2).

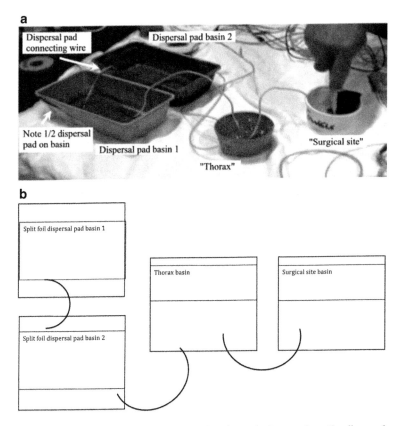

Fig. 21.1. (**a**) Actual model of a head and neck surgical case where the dispersal pad is placed on the thigh or buttock, creating a presumed current path through the thorax. Note the split foil dispersive pad has been cut in half and placed on two metal basins, which are filled with a saline-water-ultrasonic gel solution and connected together with a bridge wire to create appropriate impedance for the dispersal site skin integrity monitor on the ES generator. (**b**) Schematic drawing of model with presumed current path from the "surgical site" through the "thorax" to the "dispersal pad site." The *black lines* represent insulated 12-gauge copper wire with insulation stripped off 5–10 cm on both ends, which were placed into the liquid baths as described in the text.

Creation of Electromagnetic Interference (EMI)

To evaluate the creation of EMI, the hand tool was applied to the green towel remnant in the "surgical site" basin, either directly, via a hemostat (instrument approach), or allowed to spark while operating the

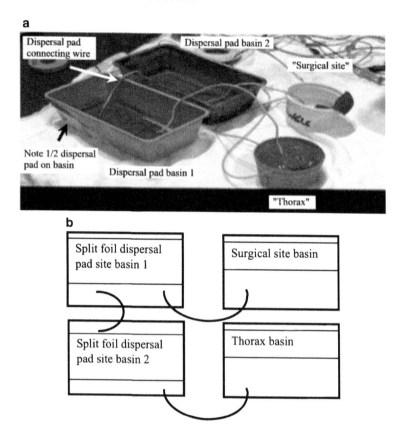

Fig. 21.2. (**a**) Actual model of a surgical case where the dispersal pad is placed to prevent the presumed current path from crossing the thorax. This model simulates a typical pelvic case with the dispersal pad on the thigh or buttock, or a head and neck case with the dispersal pad on the posterior-superior shoulder contralateral to the CIED generator. Note the split foil dispersive pad has been cut in half and placed on two metal basins, which are filled with a saline-water-ultrasonic gel solution and connected together with a bridge wire to create appropriate impedance for the dispersal site skin integrity monitor on the ES generator. (**b**) Schematic drawing of model with presumed current path from the "surgical site" to the "dispersal pad site" without passing through the "thorax." The *black lines* represent insulated 12-gauge copper wire with insulation stripped off 5–10 cm on both ends, which were placed into the liquid baths as described in the text.

hand tool. The programmed values were chosen to identify EMI (1) entering on the ventricular channel, which causes the CIED to "believe" that the ventricle has spontaneous electrical activity and needs no pacing support. With the CIED set to pace at 70 bpm (which would create wide complex QRS) and the PHS set to 40 bpm (which would create narrow complex QRS), ventricular-sensed EMI would be recognized as a fall in ECG rate from 75 to 40 bpm with the appearance of narrow complex QRS. The CIEDs used in this simulation also have the ability to record these high-frequency ventricular-sensed events for later review; and (2) entering on the atrial channel, which will cause the CIED to "believe" that the atrium has high-frequency depolarizations. The CIED will enter "mode switch" to prevent tracking of this high atrial rate into the ventricle. It will pace VVI (ventricular only) at 100 bpm, so the ECG signal will increase to a rate of 100 bpm and the QRS complexes will remain wide. The CIEDs used in this simulation also have the ability to record these high-frequency atrial-sensed events for later review.

The ECG revealed several patterns:

1. No change from 75 bpm, AVd 180 ms, LBBB pattern QRS (no EMI)→all pacing initiated by the CIED and no EMI signals detected on the electrodes in the "thorax" basin.
2. Change to 40 bpm, AVd 300 ms, narrow complex QRS→EMI was presumed to enter the system on the ventricular CIED channel, thus inhibiting both atrial and ventricular output from the CIED, returning the "patient" to their original rhythm.
3. Change to 100 bpm, LBBB pattern→presumed EMI entering the atrial channel, which CIED interprets as atrial fibrillation and changes pacing to the atrial fibrillation mode. There will be no atrial pacing in this mode.
4. Change to 75 bpm, AVd 300 ms, narrow complex QRS→(this is perplexing). Either EMI interfered with the detection of the "paced" ventricular event by the PHS, or EMI must have entered the ventricular channel intermittently, since a rate of 75 bpm is possible only if the CIED initiates the atrial event. In this case, the PHS must have sensed the atrial event created by the CIED, and since no paced ventricular event took place, the PHS then fired the ventricle at 300 ms. If EMI entered the ventricular channel continuously, then atrial output should have been inhibited (see 2, above).

5. No ECG signal, implying that EMI is affecting the PHS or the monitor. EMI affecting the monitor can be observed in the operating room, especially with ES devices like an argon beam coagulator.
6. Any combination of above.

Interrogation of the CIED after a no-change situation revealed no noise detected on either the atrial or ventricular channels. Interrogation after many of the other events revealed EMI noise on both channels.

Items observed:

1. In general, EMI is unpredictable and can occur in any configuration of the ES generator and current pathways.
2. Activation of the monopolar device without connection to any part of the "patient" increased the likelihood of EMI regardless of the ES generator output setting mode (coag, blend or cut).
3. EMI was greater in the model that passed ES current through the "thorax" basin.
4. EMI was greatest with a monopolar instrument on the "coag" ES setting. EMI decreased in the following manner.
    (a) coag > blend 3 > blend 2 > blend 1 > cut.
5. EMI was rare with a bipolar instrument (although at 80 J inserting the bipolar hand tool into the "thorax" basin created considerable EMI upon activation).
6. EMI increased with increasing ES power output, sometimes affecting the monitor or the patient simulator.
7. EMI was greater when the monopolar device was applied to an instrument holding the towel in the "surgical site" basin.
8. EMI was greater when the monopolar device was allowed to spark against the "surgical site" towel (partly out of the basin), which appeared to mimic skin-edge application and created electrical sparks.

22. Hands-on Station: Radiofrequency Electrosurgery in Gastrointestinal Endoscopy

Jeffrey W. Hazey

Objectives

1. Understand the fundamentals of monopolar, bipolar, and argon plasma coagulation (APC) devices as they apply to flexible instrumentation.
2. Understand the unique depth of penetration of the various modalities.
3. Reconstruct the simulation for education and "hands-on" learning.

Introduction

This simulation outlines the basic use of radiofrequency energy delivered by different flexible instruments through a flexible endoscope. Instruments routinely used for upper and lower endoscopic therapy include monopolar, bipolar, and APC devices. Due to the long distance (i.e., the electrode is on the end of a flexible instrument and remote to the hands of the operator), activation of energy is performed via a foot pedal. The end effect of "coag", "blend" or pure "cut" settings, is determined visually without haptic feedback. In this hands-on simulation model, the unique characteristics of monopolar, bipolar, and APC devices will be highlighted for clinical application. In this module, visual evaluation of the effects of radiofrequency energy on the luminal and extraluminal surfaces of tissue is paramount since it occurs remotely. The equipment list is included so that the module can be reconstructed for learning. While specific vendors are suggested to reproduce the setup, other vendors of comparable instruments may certainly be used.

L.S. Feldman et al. (eds.), *The SAGES Manual on the Fundamental Use of Surgical Energy (FUSE)*, DOI 10.1007/978-1-4614-2074-3_22, © Springer Science+Business Media, LLC 2012

Equipment List

Vendor	Equipment
Olympus	Video tower
	Water bottle for irrigation
	Suction tubing with suction capabilities (cannister)
	Diagnostic gastroscope (single channel)
	Dispersive ("Grounding") pad (REM polyhesive II) E7507
	Hot biopsy FD-230U
	Snare SD-210U-25
	Solar probe CD-B420LA+adaptor
	IT knife 2 KD-611C
	Hookknife KD-611C
	Flexknife KD-630L
	Triangle tip knife KD-640C
	Dual knife KD-650L
ERBE	Model V/O 300D 2 with argon gas
	Black adaptor for bipolar
	Side fire APC—20132-217
	Straight fire APC—20132-214
	Circumferential fire APC 20132-186
ValleyLab	Active cord 58431
DeLegge Medical	Porcine gastric explants and stabilization boards
Boston Scientific	Snare #6267
	Needle knife 4584
	Hot biopsy 1550
	Gold probe—6015+adaptor
Cook Medical	Snare AS-1G22192
	Hot biopsy G31584
	Quicksilver G24926 + adaptor

Construction of Module

This module is constructed using the equipment list provided previously. Principles outlined in this module can be applied to both lower and upper endoscopy but for ease, a porcine gastric explant and standard gastroscope is used to outline these principles (Fig. 22.1). The gastric implant is secured on a peg board with a grounding pad in contact with the posterior wall of the stomach between the explant and peg board. A standard endoscopic tower with suction and an irrigation bottle is positioned at a comfortable distance beside the explant. Water soluble

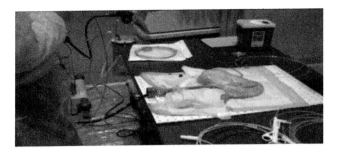

Fig. 22.1. Principles outlined in this module can be applied to both lower and upper endoscopy, but for this example, a porcine gastric explant and standard gastroscope is used to outline these principles.

lubricant is needed to facilitate passage of the endoscope through the esophageal opening reinforced with a plastic insert in the proximal esophagus. Passage of the flexible endoscope allows access to the explant esophagus, stomach, and duodenum. Each of the three devices (monopolar, bipolar, and APC) is delivered to the three anatomically different parts of the explant to highlight the unique characteristics (i.e., thickness) of the esophagus, stomach, and duodenum. External visualization with application of energy allows the endoscopist/student to understand depth of penetration and tissue effects of different energy modalities. Similarly, use of multiple instruments to deliver energy allows the endoscopist to see their unique effects on the serosal or extraluminal side of the explant to illustrate safety. The endoscopist is encouraged to apply energy settings used clinically and test the limits of energy application. The purpose is to provide the endoscopist a safe venue to see how much energy and force is required to perforate or create a full thickness injury with the energy sources at their disposal. Visualization of the extraluminal side of the organ is essential so the endoscopist is aware of potential pitfalls.

Monopolar Instruments

Endoscopic application of radiofrequency energy using monopolar devices follows standard principles used in the operating room with other monopolar devices. The active electrode at the tip of the flexible instrument has a small contact area with high current density to create the desired thermal effect. As with other monopolar devices, placement of the dispersive pad is essential for safe use. Good tissue apposition across a broad base ensures low current density to avoid undesired thermal injury. Contact area with the patient must be uniform over a large surface area. Bony prominences, metal implants, scar tissue, hairy areas, etc. should be avoided. Radiofrequency energy is applied with a number of different flexible monopolar instruments with differing purposes. Of the three energy devices outlined in this module, depth of penetration is greatest with monopolar devices and varies with the amount of current applied, the time the current is applied, and the resistance of the tissue to which it is applied.

1. A monopolar "hot" biopsy forceps is used to biopsy tissue that possesses the potential for bleeding. Biopsy can be performed "cold" (i.e., without the use of energy) when architecture of the tissue wishes to be maintained for pathologic analysis. The use of electrosurgery can alter the cellular architecture and make histological evaluation of the lesion in question difficult. Thus, the use of energy in conjunction with biopsy should be reserved for the clinical scenario when histology is not essential or bleeding is a significant risk. As with all energy devices, the mucosa should be elevated away from the submucosal before applying energy to the lesion in question to prevent deeper penetration.

2. Snares are typically used to resect polyps or perform endoscopic mucosal resection (EMR) of polypoid (sessile or pedunculated) lesions. Different types of currents are applied to the snare to show the different tissue effects. Injection of submucosal saline can protect the submucosa from thermal injury and is often recommended when resecting sessile polyps or non-polypoid mucosal lesions. As with hot biopsy forceps, elevation of the mucosa away from the submucosal is essential to limit submucosal exposure to electrical current and prevent a full thickness injury.

3. A number of other flexible instruments are available to facilitate tissue dissection and/or cutting for a wide variety of clinical applications. Configurations vary all with the purpose of facilitating delivery of energy in unique circumstances. The needle knife may be used to cut tissue to facilitate ERCP as in a pre-cut sphincterotomy. An IT (insulation-tip), hook, or flex knife may be used to cut/coagulate tissue during submucosal dissection. Familiarity of these instruments is essential so that they may be used for the desired effect in the appropriate clinical setting.

Bipolar Instruments

The use of bipolar instruments during flexible endoscopy is generally reserved for hemostasis as the application of energy is more controlled with less tissue penetration than with monopolar devices. As the name implies, the tip of the flexible instrument possesses both electrodes so that current flows solely between the electrodes. The safety profile is improved with these devices in order to prevent full thickness tissue destruction and potential perforation.

Bipolar probes "(e.g., Gold Probe™ (Boston Scientific), Quicksilver® (Cook Medical)) are most often used for hemostasis. The probes provides the endoscopist with the ability to inject and irrigate, facilitating hemostasis with one instrument. As part of the module, application of energy to the mucosal surface of the esophagus, stomach, and duodenum with this device illustrates the relative shallow penetration of current with an improved safety profile.

Argon Plasma Coagulation

The application of radiofrequency energy via a "beam" of argon gas offers the endoscopist the ability to fulgurate/ablate superficial mucosal lesions/pathology with the least/lowest depth of penetration among the energy devices discussed in this module. This is essentially a monopolar energy device with current transmitted through a gaseous environment rather than physical contact. Depth of penetration is limited to just a few millimeters making APC uniquely suited for superficial mucosal tissue destruction. It typically is used for wide areas of tissue ablation including superficial vascular pathologies (i.e., AVMs) and proctitis. Argon gas is dispersed through a hollow flexible instrument in an orientation determined by the tip of the instrument. The pattern of current delivery can be straight through a hollow end or deflected to the side depending on the location and orientation of the tissue to be affected relative to the end of the endoscope. Circumferential catheters allow for dispersion of gas and current in 360° that is uniquely suited for endoluminal ablative therapies. This module is designed to highlight the different ablation catheters and their depth of penetration. Endoscopists are alerted to the fact that argon gas is being infused into the hollow viscous and when coupled with persistent insufflation can cause overdistension requiring the endoscopist to be sensitive to decompression of the hollow viscous when using this technique (Fig. 22.2).

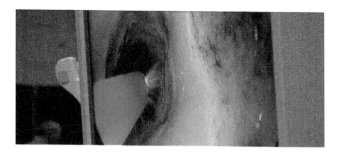

Fig. 22.2. Argon gas infused into the hollow viscous and coupled with persistent insufflation can cause overdistension, requiring the endoscopist to be sensitive to decompression of the hollow viscous when using this technique.

Fundamentals and Safety

Monopolar energy devices
Component: *Generator settings.*
Equipment: ESU, foot pedal, monopolar cord for monopolar endoscopic instruments, "hot" biopsy forceps, snare, additional monopolar instruments (IT knife, hook knife, needle knife).
Exercise: Demonstrate ESU components, jacks, displays, and controls in the context of a circuit with various monopolar instruments.

Bipolar energy devices
Component: *Generator settings.*
Equipment: ESU, foot pedal, bipolar cord for bipolar endoscopic instruments, bipolar probes.
Exercise: Demonstrate ESU components, jacks, displays, and controls in the context of a circuit with various bipolar instruments.

Argon plasma coagulation
Component: *Generator settings including rate of gas flow.*
Equipment: ESU with argon gas source, foot pedal, straight fire, side fire, and circumferential fire catheters.
Exercise: Demonstrate ESU components, jacks, displays, controls, use of circumferential fire APC in the esophagus, side fire APC in the esophagus, and duodenum and straight fire APC in the stomach.

Appendix

Energy Terms and Definitions

Preferred	Description	Alternate	Abbreviation/ Acronym	Avoid
Radiofrequency (RF) electrosurgical generator	Device, usually in a box-shaped format, used to convert wall outlet frequency (60 Hz) to radiofrequency (approx. 300–3,500 kHz) and for the control of output waveform and voltage. Most ESUs operate between 300 and 500 kHz	Electrosurgical unit	ESU	Bovie, cautery machine, Bovie-cautery machine, Bovie unit, etc.
Active electrode	Electrodes designed with a small surface area that facilitates the creation of a zone of high current (power) density and the resulting creation of a thermally based surgical effect. Monopolar instruments have only an active electrode; bipolar instruments have both electrodes. Typically, but not always, both of these are designed to function as active electrodes	Could consider terms such as "functional" electrode, "surgical" electrode, "focused" electrode" but they seem cumbersome		Bovie, Bovie pencil, etc.
Dispersive electrode	The large surface-area electrode, usually used in conjunction with monopolar instruments, that completes the circuit, but which "defocuses" the energy thereby preventing thermal injury at the site of attachment. In some instances, a dispersive electrode will be built into a bipolar instrument	N/A		Ground pad, return electrode, passive electrode, neutral electrode, indifferent electrode

(continued)

L.S. Feldman et al. (eds.), *The SAGES Manual on the Fundamental Use of Surgical Energy (FUSE)*, DOI 10.1007/978-1-4614-2074-3, © Springer Science+Business Media, LLC 2012

(continued)

Preferred	Description	Alternate	Abbreviation/ Acronym	Avoid
Monopolar instrument	A surgical instrument designed for vaporization/cutting, coagulation/desiccation, and/or fulguration with only one active electrode	Unipolar instrument		Monopolar energy, Bovie device, cautery stick
Bipolar instrument	A surgical instrument usually designed for coagulation/desiccation, but occasionally for vaporization/cutting, with two electrodes. When designed for coagulation/desiccation, both electrodes are generally "active." When designed for vaporization/cutting, one electrode is generally	N/A		Bipolar energy, any proprietary term such as "Kleppinger," "PK," etc.
Vaporization	The process whereby intracellular temperature is rapidly elevated to 100°C resulting in a liquid–gas conversion and the generation of steam. The massive expansion of volume results in rupture of the cell wall, releasing the now gaseous cellular contents. This process is most easily achieved with a thin or narrow monopolar instrument			Cautery
Desiccation	The process of loss of intracellular water secondary to cellular heating. This occurs at temperatures in excess of 45 but less than 100. The latter circumstance would result in the formation of steam and, consequently, cellular vaporization. It is likely that this process is facilitated by thermal damage to the cellular membrane. It typically occurs in conjunction with protein coagulation. Desiccation can be created with either monopolar or bipolar instruments	Dehydration		Cautery

(continued)

(continued)

Preferred	Description	Alternate	Abbreviation/ Acronym	Avoid
Coagulation	Actually protein coagulation, and sometimes called "white coagulation." The process occurs, typically above 50° but below 100° with the rupture and random reformation of intracellular hydrothermal bonds. This process occurs in conjunction with cellular dehydration or desiccation, and is typically exploited to seal blood vessels to maintain or attain hemostasis. This type of coagulation can be created with monopolar or bipolar instruments	White coagulation		Cautery
Fulguration	Also called "black coagulation." A type of superficial protein coagulation created by the establishment of an array of current arcs in the gap between the electrode and the underlying tissue. Fulguration requires the use of modulated high voltage waveforms typically produced by the "coagulation" output of the electrosurgical generator and a "no touch" technique. Tissue temperatures become higher than with either vaporization or "white coagulation" typically exceeding 200°C and resulting in organic molecular breakdown and carbonization. Fulguration is most effective for superficial coagulation and desiccation of superficial, capillary and small arteriolar bleeding ("ooze")	Black coagulation; spray coagulation		Cautery

(continued)

(continued)

Preferred	Description	Alternate	Abbreviation/ Acronym	Avoid
"Cutting" waveform	A misnomer that describes a continuous relatively low voltage waveform generated by the electrosurgical unit that appears as a "sine wave" on an oscilloscope. When there is no modulation of this output (100% duty cycle) it is often called "pure cut." The misnomer refers to the fact that this is the preferred waveform for electrosurgical desiccation and coagulation, particularly for sealing blood vessels	Low voltage current		Cautery
"Coagulation" waveform	A misnomer that describes a modulated, high voltage, but dampened (progressively reduced amplitude) waveform that typically has a duty cycle of less than 10%. This waveform can be used for fulguration, and can be useful for vaporization/cutting in high impedance situations. It is not suitable for blood vessel sealing because of the inhomogeneous and superficial nature of the resulting coagulation	High voltage current	"Coag"	Cautery
"Blended" waveforms	A misnomer that suggests mixing of two outputs. "Blend" waveforms are actually modulated (but not dampened) low voltage outputs from the "cut" side of the ESU. The duty cycle of these outputs is typically between 30 and 80%, with the peak voltage rising as the duty cycle reduces. These waveforms are designed to provide an increased amount of protein coagulation beside an electrosurgical incision	Modulated low voltage current	"Blend"	Cautery

(continued)

(continued)

Preferred	Description	Alternate	Abbreviation/ Acronym	Avoid
Duty cycle	The proportion of time that a waveform is being generated per unit time. Duty cycles can range from about 6% for the high voltage ("coag") outputs to 100% in the "pure cut" waveforms			
Power density	The amount of power delivered to a given area of tissue. The higher the power density, the greater the potential for cellular and tissue heating. Power density and current density are actually different calculations, but both reflect the amount of energy delivered to a given site per unit time. Very low power densities are associated with no tissue effect (example dispersive electrode), moderately high power densities allow tissue heating adequate to desiccate and coagulate; while high power densities result in vaporization of the cell and tissue			
Power	The amount of energy consumed per unit time; it is a product of voltage (V) and current (I) and is measured in Watts (see Watts)		P	
Direct current	Current produced by an electrical circuit that is the product of an energy source with constant polarity. On an oscilloscope, the deflection of the display is either constantly above or below "0" to a degree that reflects the voltage in the circuit		DC	

(continued)

(continued)

Preferred	Description	Alternate	Abbreviation/ Acronym	Avoid
Alternating current	Current produced by an electrical circuit that results from an energy source with continuously changing polarity. On an oscilloscope, the wave traverses above and below "0" reflecting the changing polarity. The frequency of the change in polarity is expressed in hertz (Hz) with 1 Hz = 1 full cycle per second		AC	
Current	The flow of electrons past or across a given point in the circuit per unit time and is measured in Amperes (see Ampere)		I	
Impedance	The amount of impairment of electron or ionic flow (current) imparted by a given substance that forms part of an alternating polarity (alternating current) circuit		R	
Resistance	The amount of impairment of electron or ionic flow (current) imparted by a given substance that forms part of a constant polarity (direct current) circuit		R	
Current density	The amount of current per unit of cross-sectional area passing through a circuit. It is analogous to but not the same as power density. Very low current densities are associated with no tissue effect (e.g., dispersive electrode), moderately high current densities allow tissue heating adequate to desiccate and coagulate, while high current densities result in vaporization of the cell and tissue			
Watt	An expression of power; 1 W = 1 J/s		W	

(continued)

Preferred	Description	Alternate	Abbreviation/ Acronym	Avoid
Joule	A unit of energy that really reflects the capacity to perform work. One Joule = 1 W/s			
Ampere	A measure of the movement of ions in a circuit, or current (I). 1 A−1 C/s		Amp	
Ohm	A measure of electrical resistance (in a direct current circuit) or of impedance (in an alternating polarity circuit). Biological tissue requires high water and ionic content to have the least resistance. Tissue such as fat, scar tissue, or electrosurgically desiccated tissue has relatively high impedance		R	
Volt, voltage	The difference in electrical potential between two points in a circuit, that is expressed in volts (V)		V	
Radiofrequency	Refers to the frequency of the electromagnetic spectrum that ranges between 300 kHz and 3 MHz. Most surgical RF electrosurgical generators generate frequencies of 400–500 kHz		RF	
Open circuit	A situation that occurs when the electrosurgical generator is activated when the circuit is not complete. For example, in the operating room, the ESU is activated when the active electrode is not near to or in contact with tissue			

Index